Peptides Are Life

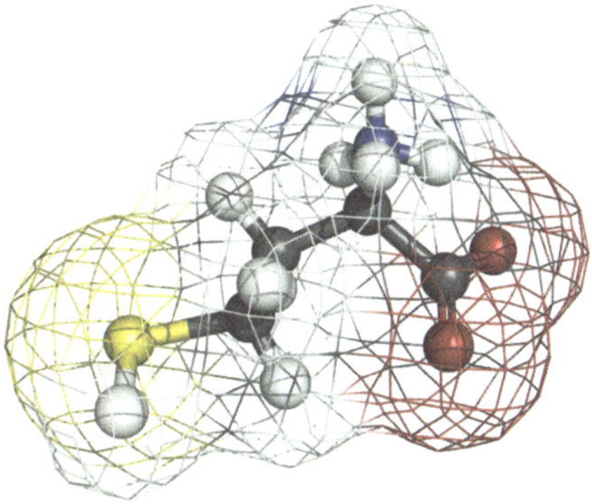

LAURISTON CROCKETT III
ACCREDITED HEALTH AND WELLNESS EXPERT

HIS Publishing Group
4301 Wiley Post Road
Suite 201D
Addison, TX 75001

Library of Congress Control Number: 2021907988

Peptides are Life: Lauriston Crockett III a recognized expert in protein peptide technologies provides an in depth and easy to understand approach for those looking to improve longevity and body rejuvenation.

1. Health and Fitness 2. Medical 3. Science

ISBN: 978-1-7370247-0-5 *paperback*
978-1-7370247-1-2 *ebook*

Printed in the United States of America
First Edition

HIS PUBLISHING GROUP
Division of Human Improvement Specialists llc.
www.hispubg.com | *info@hispubg.com*

Acknowledgement

I wanted to give a special thank you to

Mr. Thomas Lima, Mr. Jeff Shaffer
and Mr. Kevin Rachel

Your confidence in this project and
friendship means the world to me.

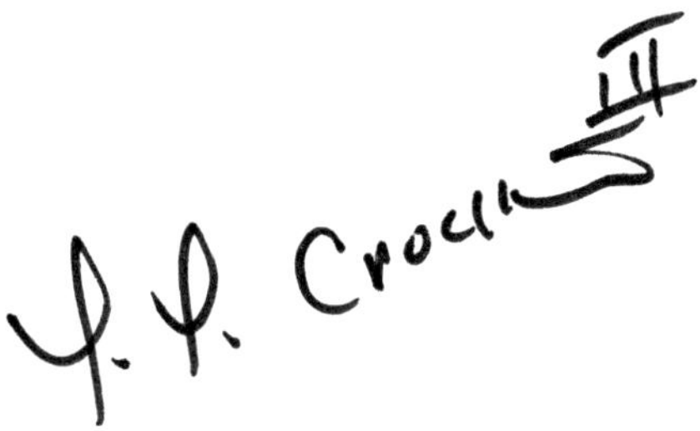

Dedication

I wrote this book in dedication to my young son,

Lauriston Crockett IV

I love you and may you live until
one hundred and ten.

Table of Contents

Introduction

Peptides Are Life

"Peptides, part of the essential building blocks of life, are an important field of study and those involved in this field continue making new discoveries.". Researchers carry on with documenting an ever-expanding list of capabilities and benefits of peptides. Farmers are applying them to increase the yields of their crops. Bodybuilders are using them to boost strength and endurance. Cosmetic companies promise they will produce smoother, younger-looking skin. Exciting new research strongly suggests that they may slow aging at the cellular level and strengthen the body's defenses against disease-causing organisms like bacteria and viruses.

What Is A Peptide?

The word peptide comes from the Greek word, peptós, meaning, "digested." After you eat a juicy hamburger, tasty chicken breast, or other Protein-rich food, your body begins to break down these proteins into their basic structure of amino acids.

These amino acids are peptides. Peptides consist of chains of anywhere from two to fifty amino acids. These amino acids are compounds constructed from nitrogen, oxygen, carbon, and hydrogen: the essential building blocks of all life. The process of digestion ultimately makes these vital molecules available for utilization by all the cells of your body to sustain life and health.

As you can see in the figure below, amino acids are separate groups of different molecules until they are forged into a peptide chain.

How your body uses amino acids as building blocks

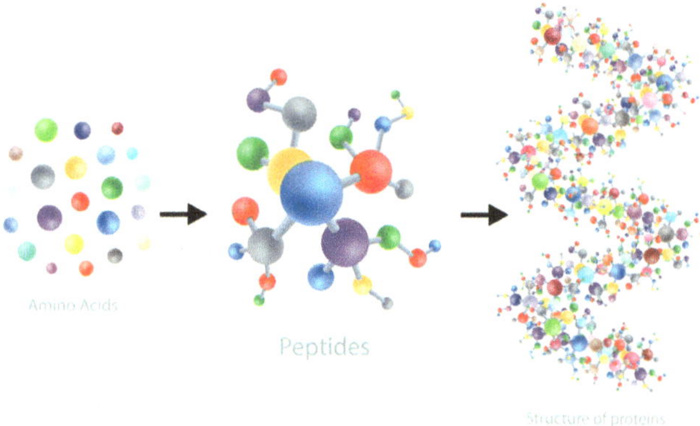

This happens when one group of amino acids is joined to another by a chemical reaction that binds them together, called the peptide bond. The resulting chains of peptides may be short or long. A short chain consisting of only two amino acids is a dipeptide, while a chain composed of many amino acids is called a polypeptide ("poly" means many). A protein combines long chains of polypeptides and usually consists of fifty or more amino acids. However, the line between peptides and proteins is often blurred, and sources also describe some polypeptides as "small proteins."

Why Are Peptides Important To Life?

Regardless, if peptides are assembled into larger proteins or broken down into amino acids, they play a crucial role in the human body and often have varying applications Some peptides, called signaling molecules, transmit information between cells and cause specific reactions and changes inside the cells that receive the signal. In the brain, these "peptide-signaling" molecules are called neuropeptides, and they activate communication between neurons, or brain cells. At least 100 known neuropeptides regulate critical brain functions, including pain relief, appetite, learning, and memory.

Another one of the one hundred known neuropeptides is the growth factor. Not to be confused with growth hormones, growth factors are forms of peptide signaling molecules which regulate the growth, development, and the proliferation of cells. In fact, there are several major families of growth factors. Of those, important ones to note include polypeptides, which stimulate the growth and development of healthy animal and human fetuses, and others which help repair and heal wounds and even regulate the survival and death of cells.

Researchers around the world are investigating the many potential therapeutic applications of growth factors in the restoration and regeneration of injured tissues. For example, a growing number of clinical studies have demonstrated that some growth factors can repair skin which has been damaged by the sun and significantly diminish the appearance of lines, wrinkles, and other signs of aging. Another important class of peptides, called cationic host defense peptides or host defense peptides (HDPs), help fight bacteria, viruses, fungi, and parasites. They were traditionally called antimicrobial peptides (AMPs) however, researchers have discovered that host defense peptides perform a wider array of functions than just combating or defending against microbes. They can boost the body's innate immune response and possess wound-healing and anti-inflammatory properties. The antimicrobial properties may even make them crucial weapons in fighting antibiotic-resistant bacteria and viruses like the new coronavirus, SARS-CoV-2. Unfortunately, peptides do not exist without obstacles that can impede their ability to function. One such disorder is Type 1 diabetes. With Type I diabetes, the pancreas fails to manufacture a peptide hormone, insulin, which is crucial to the regulation of the levels of glucose or sugar in the blood. Nearly 100 years ago, scientists discovered the first effective pharmaceutical treatment for this disease: injections of an extract made from a cow pancreas to replace the missing insulin.

Animal insulin can be sourced from a pig or cows' pancreas. The Insulin would then be purified to help the user from developing any reaction. Animal insulins have been developed into 3 different types. "short acting, intermediate and long acting"

Discovery Of Peptides: Diabetes And Insulin

Doctors have been familiar with the deadly disease called diabetes for thousands of years. The disorder causes too much glucose, or sugar, to accumulate in the bloodstream, resulting in damage to internal organs. This damage can go on to cause severe health problems, many of which routinely prove fatal without effective treatment. The first known written reference to diabetes dates back to an Egyptian papyrus from about 1552 B.C. Additionally, until the twentieth century, children born with Type 1 diabetes tended to live short, miserable lives. Those who developed diabetes later in life, also had a bleak prognosis. The link between diabetes and the pancreas was established in the late nineteenth century. Many researchers experimented with pancreatic extracts, but trials of the extracts in human patients usually failed due to harmful side-effects. In 1921, Frederick G. Banting, J.J.R. Macleod, and Charles Best tried a different approach to obtaining the extract from the islet cells. "Islets are cells found in clusters in the pancreas". Biochemist James Bertram Collip later joined them in Macleod's laboratory in Toronto,

Canada, to assist with the work of producing a purified extract which could be used in clinical trials on humans.

In January 1922, the new compound was injected into Leonard Thompson, a fourteen-year-old diabetic boy who weighed only sixty-five pounds when admitted to the hospital. By the next day, the patient's blood glucose dropped significantly. His symptoms and appearance improved, and he felt better. He lived thirteen more years using the new treatment. Six more patients were treated successfully the following month. The Toronto team named the extract "insuline" in a paper they published in April 1922. Millions of people around the world have lived longer, healthier lives ever since the team's ground-breaking work on this crucial peptide hormone. The discovery of insulin led to the identification of other peptides that play key roles in the regulation of blood sugar, such as glucagon and somatostatin. The work of the Toronto team was just the beginning of what would become the scientific explorations of peptides and their amazing potential for both medical research and the development of numerous therapeutic agents and nutritional formulas.

Peptides' Unique Potential For Research And Pharmaceuticals

Scientific understanding of peptides is less than a century old, and the pace of inquiry into these essential building blocks of life continues to accelerate. Recent research has yielded highly promising results and intriguing new directions for further investigation. Growth factors demonstrate great potential for the repair and healing of wounds and burns. Researchers are reporting substantial rejuvenating effects from peptide formulas, including new collagen formation, improvements in skin thickness and texture, and reductions in the depth of lines and wrinkles. The future of these innovative cosmeceuticals looks bright as they are becoming popular alternatives to invasive and expensive surgical procedures.

It is clear that in many respects, biochemists have only just begun to unravel the mysteries and potentials of peptides.

In Chapter one, we will examine some specific peptides in greater detail and learn more about their critical functions in human life, health, and behavior. Chapter two will explore the different ways our bodies naturally obtain these vitally important compounds.

Fortunately, biomedical researchers have formulated peptide compounds which can supplement or replace the natural sources. Our review of the history of pharmaceutical applications of peptides will begin in Chapter three with the Soviet Union, which pioneered peptide technology in the 1980s. Chapter four will explore modern peptide science.

Chapter five explores the action and impacts of the two main families of Host Defense Peptides (HDPs) defensins and cathelicidins.

Chapter six examines the history, development, and science of the revolutionary Genostim® Hexatide™ Peptide. This unique peptide contains twenty-one naturally occurring growth factors which make up the key bioactive components in all Genostim® compounds. We will examine each of the specific growth factors in Genostim®'s extracts and the medical science behind their rejuvenating effects at a cellular level.

The book concludes in Chapter seven with an overview of the future of peptide science and the many potential clinical applications of these biomolecules. Researchers continue making new discoveries about the profound biological impacts and potential health benefits of biopeptides, and Genostim® Performance Labs' science and technology will be on the cutting edge of these exciting developments.

~

Let's dive in and look at some specific peptides and their fascinating impacts on human life and health. Can you build up your immune system to fight dangerous diseases, even new microbial threats such as COVID-19? Is there a way to rejuvenate your body on a cellular level and restore youthful vitality and vigor?

Peptides could be the key!

Chapter One

Bioactive Peptides: Cellular Communicators, Defenders, and Rejuvenators

Bioactive peptides are small, but their physiological effects are enormous. So far, over 7,000 peptides have been identified in nature, and they are at the center of many of our most fundamental physical needs, emotions, and behaviors. Neuropeptides in the brain transmit messages between neurons, or brain cells. These communications profoundly impact process such as food intake, learning and memory, and the sensation of pain. Antimicrobial peptides and Host Defense Peptides, or HDPs, are essential to the effective mobilization of your body's internal defenses against external threats such as pathogens and parasites. Growth factors including GHK-Cu, or copper peptide, stimulate the repair and regeneration of all the cells and tissues in your body.

Your Body's Cellular Communications Network: Peptides As Signaling Molecules

All the cells in your body are constantly communicating with each other. Their signals, or messages, are transmitted in the form of molecules called ligands. Successful transmission of the signal initiates a response in the target cell. This successful transmission occurs when ligands attach to a cell at a precise location, called a receptor. It is similar to a key fitting into a lock. Ligands also known as Signaling molecules can take a wide variety of forms, including ions, small proteins, and peptides.

Signaling molecules travel to their destinations via four signals paracrine, endocrine, autocrine, and direct. Paracrine signals are transmitted to nearby cells, and they cause rapid but brief responses. Endocrine signals are produced by endocrine cells such as the thyroid and pituitary glands. These ligands called hormones, travel some distance through the bloodstream to reach the target cells and cause slower but longer-lasting effects. Autocrine ("auto" meaning "self") signals regulate pain sensation and anti-inflammatory responses and can be released by a cell and even act upon the cell itself. Direct signals are transmitted to a neighboring cell through small channels that connect their cell membranes. Large proteins cannot pass through the channels, so ligands are often calcium ions or small molecules like peptides. Depending upon the specific ligands and cell receptors, the target cell responds to these signals in a variety of different ways. The cell's response often includes internal changes that can affect the cell's metabolic processes or promote cell growth or cell death.

Looking at the brain specifically, cell-to-cell communication in the brain is carried out by signaling molecules. These signaling molecules are called neurotransmitters, which take three major forms: peptides, amino acids, and monoamines. The peptide neurotransmitters are neuropeptides which help regulate the increase or decrease of synaptic signaling. A wide range of neuropeptides, peptide hormones, and growth factors function as signaling molecules in humans. They often are linked with each other through direct signaling pathways, or interact with each other, or with other chemical messengers such as monoamines, in complex ways.

Intercellular Communications In The Brain And Beyond: Neuropeptides

Neuropeptides transmit messages between neurons which are the cells of the brain. These messages, or signals, can cause changes inside the cells that receive them, often stimulating a cascade of downstream signals with additional effects. Currently at least 100 neuropeptides and their receptors have been identified. These 100 neuropeptides are linked to having distinctive effects on brain and bodily functions and processes as well as human emotions and behaviors. Some neuropeptides regulate hunger, eating, and metabolic processes. Others relieve pain and reduce bodily stress. These applications have prompted new research and suggest that some neuropeptides could have anti-aging and life-extending effects. This is important because peptides produced in the brain clearly have powerful impacts elsewhere in your body, and chemical messengers released in other parts of your body have potent effects on the neuropeptides in your brain.

For example, a region of your brain called the hypothalamus manufactures a neuropeptide called Melanin-Concentrating Hormone (MCH). MCH activates receptors in your stomach that generate feelings of hunger, thus alerting you to eat. In 2017, researchers discovered that another neuropeptide produced in the hypothalamus, FLP-7, also referred to as "Flip 7", activates a receptor in intestinal cells that begins turning stored body fat into energy. Additionally, this same neuropeptide impacts the production of the peptide hormone known as ghrelin, produced by the cells of your gastrointestinal tract. Ghrelin stimulates the release of Neuropeptide Y in your brain, which causes you to feel hungry and start looking for your next meal. Pharmaceuticals which utilize these, and other neuropeptides and their receptors may one day help people maintain a healthy body weight.

The human body also creates a neuropeptide called Opioid peptides. These peptides are manufactured in the central nervous system (CNS) and by a variety of glands, including the pituitary and adrenal glands. They are endogenous (meaning they come from within the body) opioid peptides and are comprised of three families: endorphins, enkephalins, and dynorphins. One type of endorphin, beta endorphin or β-Endorphin, has morphine-like effects and is involved in pain relief. β-endorphins bind with opioid receptors in the peripheral nervous system located throughout the body. The same receptors that bind with drugs like opium and morphine. The binding of the β-endorphins at the receptors starts a chain reaction of processes which prevents the release of a protein called substance P that is central to the transmission of pain. At the most basic level, the primary function of β-endorphins is to reduce stress and promote homeostasis or balance. For example, exercising and physical activities produce β-endorphins. In the brain this acts like a natural painkiller and reduces stress and the ability to sleep better.

Enkephalins play key roles in the cardiovascular system, gastrointestinal functions, breathing, and pain management. New research indicates enkephalins and their receptors also might improve resilience to chronic stress and promote healthy aging.

Dynorphins are thought to be involved in learning and memory, emotional control, pain, and addiction. A 2018 study identified dynorphin as a prominent participant in the neural circuits which produce anxiety. The peptide signals specific neurons in the brain which are known to produce fear responses, and the activation of those specific neurons cause higher levels of anxiety in mice. Drugs which manipulate this brain circuit on a cellular level might one day be able to alleviate anxiety caused by stress.

Many other neuropeptides are crucial to your body's homeostasis and health. Two related, similar neuropeptides, Neuropeptide W (NPW) and Neuropeptide B (NPB), are involved in a variety of physiological processes, including cardiovascular functions, hunger, eating, and the sensation of pain. For example, injections of NPW in rats dramatically increased their food intake in the short-term. However, administration of NPB in the long-term appeared to reduce excessive hunger. The NPW transmitter system has also been shown to control the body's reactions to acute pain caused by inflammation.

Neuropeptide S (NPS) appears to be powerfully involved in the formation and duration of our memories of everything from small matters to negative experiences. In tests, mice had longer, more intense recollections of learned experiences if NPS receptors in the brain were activated directly afterwards. But if the NPS receptor was disrupted, the mice's recall of the experience was weak, or they failed to remember it at all. Researchers believe that because NPS stimulates alertness while calming anxiety, it prepares the brain to learn more effectively. These discoveries could lead to new treatments for Alzheimer's disease, PTSD, and other cognitive issues.

Neuropeptide Y (NPY) is the most plentiful neuropeptide in the brain of mammals and is involved in several crucial physiological processes. Activation of a variety of different NPY receptors throughout the body results in distinctive effects, including the stimulation of hunger and food intake, regulation of cardiovascular functions, energy homeostasis, bone formation, and reduced anxiety. Therapeutic interventions targeting these receptors may hold great promise in treating metabolic disorders such as obesity.

Neuroscientists once believed that the adult brain did not create new brain cells, but that is now known to be inaccurate. Additionally, Neuropeptide Y also appears to play an important role in neurogenesis, or the creation of neurons, in various parts of the brain where cell growth and multiplication continue to occur into adulthood. This physiological function may be related to other indications that NPY plays a prominent role in aging and one's ultimate lifespan. Researchers note that transgenic rats, which have had foreign DNA incorporated in their genomes, produce excessive amounts of NPY and live longer.

Neuropeptides interact with each other and with other bioactive peptides in many complicated, synergistic ways which ultimately tend towards the maintenance of equilibrium, in the cellular environment. In some disorders, the nervous system becomes involved with immune system processes and those two functions should ultimately remain very separate for optimum functionality. Unfortunately, an example where they do not stay separated is when people who suffer brain injuries or strokes often also are stricken with severe infections such as pneumonia and urinary tract infections. These seem like separate ailments, but they can and do occur in conjunction with one another. Until recently, the reasons for this crossover remained unclear. Neuroscientists recently discovered direct pathways between the nervous system and the immune system which, when activated by a brain or spinal cord injury, resulted in a sharp decrease in the number of immune cells. Therapeutic applications which target these pathways could strengthen your entire immune system, including some of your body's fiercest defenders against infection on the cellular level: antimicrobial peptides.

Cellular Defenders: Antimicrobial Peptides

Every day, all day, our bodies are under constant attack by enemies too small to see with the naked eye: bacteria, viruses, fungi, and parasites. Fortunately, nature has developed a superb, multi-layered, defense system against these microbes, which includes bioactive peptides. They are called antimicrobial peptides (AMPs), or cationic host defense peptides (HDPs). There are at least 1,700 known antimicrobial peptides and they work with each other and with other chemical messengers to combat pathogens, or harmful organisms, and prevent infections.

When most people think of how our bodies respond to infections, they likely remember biology classes explaining the body's heroic white blood cells engulfing and destroying invading bacteria. However, that is not the entirety of the story. The tissues of our bodies also produce bioactive peptides capable of combating pathogens directly. AMPs work by puncturing the cell membrane of bacteria like a pin pops a balloon. Therefore, they offer exciting possibilities for clinical use against antibiotic-resistant bacteria. Their antimicrobial action also may be crucial to your body's ability to defend against new pathogens, such as the novel coronavirus, SARS-CoV-2.

Researchers are discovering that antimicrobial peptides also perform other key functions in restoring and maintaining bodily health. They help reduce inflammation and heal wounds and regulate the immune system's response to infection. Chapter five will deep dive into the functions of these crucial host defense peptides and their critical role in fortifying the body's Viral Shield.

Cellular Rejuvenators: Growth Factors

Growth factors are bioactive peptides which stimulate development, growth, differentiation, repair, healing, and recycling of all the cells in your body. Like other signaling molecules, they are part of the cell-to-cell communications network. They travel to the target cell, where they activate specific receptors on the surface of the cell. As explained earlier, this is like a key fitting into a lock. Growth factors include EGF (epidermal growth factor), NGF (nerve growth factor), FGF (fibroblast growth factors), CTGF (connective tissue growth factor), and TGF- β (Transforming Growth Factor-Beta). These and other growth factors currently are undergoing numerous, intensive investigations into their possibilities for repairing, regenerating, and rejuvenating damaged and aging cells, tissues, and organs.

EGF (Epidermal Growth Factor)

The first growth factor to be discovered by scientists. It is a signal to the epithelial cells that line the outer and inner surfaces of your body that they should grow, develop, or die. Epithelial tissues include your skin cells and the cells that form the outside surfaces of your intestinal tract. Cells release EGF, which either stimulates the cell's own growth, or it prompts them to divide because the EGF is absorbed by nearby cells. With its receptor, EGFR, it plays a crucial role in wound healing and tissue regeneration.

NGF (Nerve Growth Factor)

Discovered in the 1950s by an Italian neurologist, Rita Levi-Montalcini. She won a Nobel Prize for her work in 1986. NGF is a neurotrophin ("trophin" is from the Greek word for food or nutrition).

It regulates the creation, growth, differentiation, and survival of neurons, or nerve cells, as well as some types of immune cells. Researchers are investigating the potential for NGF in the treatment of brain injuries, peripheral neuropathy, and neurodegenerative disorders like Parkinson's disease. Nobel winner Levi-Montalcini claimed that she self-treated daily with eye drops containing NGF. She was 103 when she died in 2012.

FGF (Fibroblast Growth Factors)

Discovered in pituitary extracts in 1973, and it is abundant in cells and tissues throughout the body. Fibroblasts are the main cells in connective tissue. They stimulate the production of collagen and other structural components of the skin. Currently, there are twenty-two known members of the FGF family. With their receptors, (FGFRs), they control the growth, development, migration, and specialization of cells during the development of the embryo. In adults, FGFs respond to injuries and repair skin wounds by stimulating fibroblasts and angiogenesis, the creation of new blood vessels. FGS have shown exciting potential for the regeneration of tissues, including skin, muscle, bone, tendon/ligament, cartilage, blood vessel, tooth, and nerve tissues.

CTGF (Connective Tissue Growth Factor)

Originally found to induce the multiplication and migration of fibroblasts as well as the formation of the network of molecules and proteins, such as collagen, that provides the structural scaffolding of a cell. However, substantial evidence indicates that CTGF's role in the body is much more complex and extensive. It stimulates the creation and specialization of adult stem cells in bone marrow, as well as osteoblasts, the large cells that form and shape bone, and chondrocytes, the cells that produce cartilage. Due to its involvement in these processes, CTGF boosts the healing of wounds and the regeneration of cartilage and bone.

TGF-β (Transforming Growth Factor-Beta)

Like many other growth factors, TGF-β plays a variety of complex roles in the body and regulates multiple processes. TGF-β controls the production and development of skeletal tissues, cartilage, and blood vessels. It is prominent in wound healing and anti-inflammatory responses and is crucial to the process of healing bone fractures. TGF-β signals maintain tissue homeostasis throughout the body by controlling cell growth, development, and death. Modification of TGF-β signals could provide effective treatments of osteoarthritis, immune disorders, and the growth and spread of cancer.

Other Rejuvenating Peptides: GHK

The human peptide GHK was discovered in 1973, when it caused old liver cells to manufacture proteins like young liver cells. This bioactive peptide plays multiple roles in human physiological processes, and, remarkably, "all of them appear to be health positive." (Pickart, 2018).

In a compound called GHK-Cu, copper peptide, it has wound-healing, anti-inflammatory, antioxidant, anti-aging properties and is widely used in skin care products to treat and prevent facial wrinkles and lines and boost skin firmness and elasticity. It has been proven to shield skin cells from UV radiation, restore the proteins in the skin's protective barrier, increase the growth and thickness of hair, and diminish inflammation and damage caused by free radicals.

GHK-Cu's wound-healing properties have been studied extensively. It activates growth factors which stimulate blood flow to damaged skin and the creation of new blood vessels to help repair injury. It attracts white blood cells that destroy bacteria and other harmful microbes and clean up dead cells. It also draws mast cells which release proteins to close the wound and begin healing the tissues. GKH-Cu stimulates the production of collagen and elastin by skin cells and promotes the healing of bone and cartilage. In studies of mice, application of copper peptide to a scald burn resulted in enhanced blood vessel development in the burned skin and a shorter healing time.

GHK-Cu also is a potent anti-inflammatory and antioxidant compound. In several different clinical trials, researchers studied mice which had been injected with a drug to produce an inflammatory process in the lungs called fibrosis. Lung, or pulmonary, fibrosis is caused by the replacement of healthy lung tissue with connective tissue, or collagen. This process is called scarring, and it may result from diseases such as pneumonia or exposure to contaminants like asbestos. Pulmonary fibrosis in humans is a chronic, progressive, and ultimately fatal condition. The scientists found that administration of GHK-Cu significantly reduced inflammation and disrupted the signaling pathways which deposit too much collagen in lung tissues. To their surprise, copper peptide also largely reversed weight loss caused in the mice by the injection of the fibrotic drug. They concluded that GHK-Cu is a potent anti-inflammatory and antioxidant that reduces excessive deposits of collagen in the lungs and alleviates pulmonary fibrosis.

GHK-Cu also shows strong potential as an anti-aging compound. By the age of sixty, levels of copper peptide in the blood fall to less than half those seen in a twenty-year-old. The compound suppresses molecules which are believed to accelerate the aging process and supports DNA repair and the cleansing of cells. Researchers are investigating its impacts on brain functions and have found that elderly mice (twenty-eight months old) treated with GHK escaped from a maze much more quickly than geriatric mice treated with a saline solution. GHK-Cu shows amazing potential in the prevention, treatment, and improvement of age-related cognitive decline and neurodegenerative conditions such as Alzheimer's disease and Parkinson's disease.

Many bioactive peptides have been discovered only in the recent decades, and much remains to be learned about these compounds and their possible life-enhancing and life-extending benefits.

> Now that we have learned how critical the many different types of peptides are to the healthy functioning of our bodies, you may be wondering, where do they come from?
>
> How do we find these crucial compounds and acquire them for our bodies to use?

You may be surprised—and alarmed—by the answers to these questions.

Chapter Two

Where Do Bioactive Peptides Come From?

Most bioactive peptides needed for the healthy functioning of our bodies come from foods that we eat. When we eat foods containing proteins, such as meat, milk, eggs, and some grains and beans, the process of digestion breaks many of those proteins down into peptides. This process, called proteolysis, occurs when substances called enzymes are released by the pancreas into the digestive tract that chemically cut the proteins into smaller pieces. Those smaller pieces are called peptides. The peptides are "encrypted" or locked up in the protein and are biologically inactive until they are liberated from the protein by this or other hydrolyzing processes. Fermentation, cooking, and food processing can also cause the breakdown of proteins into peptides. Bioactive peptides exert their physiological effects either on local cells or tissues in the gastrointestinal tract or travel through the bloodstream and impact other body systems.

As we know, bioactive peptides consist of chains of two to fifty amino acids, the essential building blocks of all life. The type and position of the amino acids on the chain determines the peptide's structure and effects. Research indicates that shorter peptide chains possess increased bioactivity. Different sources of bioactive peptides produce different physiological impacts in the body, including antioxidant, anti-inflammatory, antimicrobial, anti-high blood pressure, anti-cancer effects, among many demonstrated health benefits. Natural sources of bioactive peptides include milk, eggs, meat, seafood, grains and other plants, fungi, and animal by-products.

Natural Sources Of Bioactive Peptides

Dairy Products

The first food-derived peptides were discovered in 1950 by a Swedish biochemist, Olof Mellander. He reported that peptides from casein, a protein in cheese, enhanced bone formation in infants suffering from rickets (a disease that weakens and softens bones in children) without additional vitamin D. Bovine (cow) dairy products like milk, cheese, and yogurt are the major sources of food-derived bioactive peptides. This is thought to result from milk's crucial role in providing nutrition to offspring after birth. Colostrum, a substance present in milk directly after childbirth, has low levels of hormones and growth factors which may play an important role in the newborn's development. Bioactive peptides are abundant in milk proteins, which are called casein proteins and whey proteins. When these proteins are processed, through digestion, fermentation, or other methods, they produce several biologically active peptides which impact the cardiovascular, nervous, and immune systems.

A well-known type of bioactive peptides found in milk proteins function as Angiotensin-Converting-Enzyme (ACE) inhibitors and thus are called antihypertensive. This means that these compounds help prevent or weaken the cellular processes that constrict blood vessels and result in higher blood pressure, called hypertension. Milk proteins release several opioid peptides with antihypertensive effects and appear to lower blood pressure without ACE inhibition.

Peptides derived from milk proteins have also demonstrated antibacterial properties, such as glycomacropeptide (GMP). Laboratory tests indicate that GMP inhibits the buildup of plaque and bacteria on tooth surfaces and thus can aid in the prevention of cavities. Lactoferricin possesses antimicrobial, antiviral, antifungal, antitumor, and anticancer properties. These peptides are also immunomodulatory, meaning they possess the ability to affect immune system processes by stimulating the production of cells like macrophages that attack and destroy microbial invaders.

Eggs

Eggs are similar to milk in that they contain many proteins which nourish the chicken embryo as it grows and develops. In addition to providing valuable sources of protein nutrition for humans, these proteins contain abundant bioactive peptides which are being studied extensively in order to determine their possible beneficial effects on human health. Peptides derived from eggs are known to affect the endocrine, nervous, immune, cardiovascular, and digestive systems.

After the peptides are liberated from the proteins in egg whites through digestion or some other form of processing, they enter the circulatory system and affect the biological activities of your body. Researchers have reported that specific egg white peptides reduce hypertension because they exercise relaxing effects on blood vessels. The egg white peptide sequence Tyr–Ala–Glu–Glu–Arg–Tyr–Pro–Ile–Leu reduced hypertension as well as acting as a powerful antioxidant because it showed high levels of activity in scavenging oxygen free radicals. Other egg peptides exercise ACE-inhibiting effects which lower blood pressure in animals and offer potential therapeutic uses in humans.

Proteins found inside a hen's egg provide not only nourishment for the developing chick, but also furnish a natural defense system against harmful microbes. One of the major egg white proteins, lysozyme, is widely used in commercial applications to kill bacteria on meat products such as sausage, salami, pork, beef, and turkey. Lysozyme also releases peptides with antimicrobial and antiviral qualities. Digestion of other egg white proteins produces peptides capable of killing bacteria like E. coli and fungi like Candida albicans.

Egg white peptides have demonstrated a number of additional beneficial impacts on human health. They have antioxidant and anticancer effects and modulate the immune system by stimulating the production of white blood cells and macrophages. Some of these peptides have been used to boost the immune system's response to cancer treatment. A peptide obtained from egg yolks has been shown to enhance the growth of bone and is called, appropriately, Bonepep.

Meat

Bioactive peptides can also be derived from the high-quality proteins found in meats such as beef, pork, chicken, and duck, and in animal by-products such as cow blood, collagen, and gelatin. After slaughter and during aging and frozen storage, meat undergoes changes that break down the proteins and release peptides. Bioactive peptides are liberated from meat products when they are cured or ripened, as when ham is dry-cured, or sausages are fermented. Peptides are also released when meat is digested in the gastrointestinal tract.

Meat peptides have demonstrated benefits for human health, including antihypertensive, antioxidant, antithrombotic, and anticancer properties.

Like milk and egg peptides, the ACE-inhibiting, blood-pressure-lowering properties of meat peptides have been the focus of intense investigation. Peptides isolated from pork and administered to rats caused large decreases in their blood pressure. Bovine collagen also furnishes ACE-inhibiting peptides. Twenty-seven peptides derived from Spanish dry-cured ham demonstrated potent antioxidant properties. Antioxidant peptides have also been isolated from pork chorizo sausages. Bioactive peptides from pork muscle have shown antithrombotic effects, meaning they reduce blood clotting, with anticoagulant effects similar to those of aspirin. Several peptides extracted from bovine proteins demonstrate the ability to destroy cancer cells and inhibit their growth.

Fish

Fish sources of bioactive peptides include tuna, sardine, herring, and salmon. The first ACE-inhibiting peptides were isolated in sardine meat in 1986 by Japanese researchers. Peptides derived from chum salmon muscle and Bigeye tuna muscle significantly lowered blood pressure in rats. Japanese scientists administered a peptide isolated from dried bonito to thirty human patients with high blood pressure or borderline hypertension. After receiving this ACE inhibitory peptide, LKPNM, for eight weeks, the test subjects' blood pressure was reduced by an average of 12 mmHg. The hydrolysate containing this peptide has been approved for inclusion in the

Foods for Specified Health Use (FOSHU) by the Ministry of Health and Welfare in Japan.

Antioxidant peptides have been isolated from a variety of fish, such as mackerel, Alaskan Pollack, tilapia, and silver carp. Purified peptide extracts from tuna dark muscle by-product scavenged 79% and 85% of oxygen free radicals and inhibited oxidation activity for more than seven days. Sturgeon muscle peptides demonstrate anti-inflammatory effects. Researchers have found bioactive peptides in a wide variety of marine sources, including squid, sea urchins, seahorses, snow crabs, shrimp, mollusks, sponges, anemones, and seaweed. Peptides derived from various species of sponges showed the capacity to destroy mouse leukemia cells in laboratory testing. Scientists are discovering that these and other marine sources yield peptides with antimicrobial, antifungal, antiviral, antithrombotic, and antitumor effects.

Plant Sources of Peptides

Plant proteins containing essential amino acids are crucial sources of nutrition for humans and animals. Only within the last two decades have scientists discovered that small peptides play a role in plant cellular signaling, and this signaling system may be one billion years old. As in animals and humans, peptides secreted by plants regulate multiple functions, including cell growth and differentiation; response to stresses such as wounding and drought; and defense against harmful organisms.

Researchers have started to extensively investigate the potential benefits of plant peptides for human health, especially because high-fat sources like meat and milk are associated with cardiovascular and metabolic diseases.

Cereals such as wheat, rice, corn, oats, sorghum, barley, rye, and millet contain carbohydrates, proteins, B-vitamins, and minerals, and supply roughly half of the energy required by the world's people every day. The top three cereals consumed by humans are wheat, rice, and corn. Peptides derived from cereal proteins have shown antihypertensive, antioxidant, and antitumor properties. Opioid peptides have been isolated from wheat gluten which may affect the gastrointestinal tract and the release of insulin.

When vegetable proteins from soybeans, chickpeas, peas, and other pulses (plant seeds) are hydrolyzed, or chemically digested by enzymes, they yield multifunctional bioactive peptides with a number of different physiological effects. In 2006, researchers isolated limenin, a plant-based peptide, from shelf-beans. It demonstrated antifungal, antibacterial, and anticancer activities. A protein extracted from chickpeas inhibited the growth of oral cancer cells without toxic effects on normal human cells. In laboratory testing, peptide fractions from soybeans have shown the ability to destroy 50% of breast and cervical cancer cells within eight hours.

Soybeans also contain opioid peptides, soymorphins, which exhibit the ability to impact multiple body systems. Soymorphin-5 reduces both anxiety and appetite. When administered orally to diabetic mice over a long period, it increased their metabolism of sugar and fats and lowered their blood sugar levels. In addition, it has demonstrated the ability to reduce appetite and food intake in hungry mice, and researchers are currently investigating its intriguing potential as a compound for weight control in humans.

Additional plant sources of bioactive peptides include pumpkins and spinach, and they are also found in a variety of other natural sources: algae, mushrooms, and edible insects. Cyclic dipeptides called DKPs are present in roasted coffee, roasted malt, cocoa, beer, aged sake, dried squid, and a beverage called chicken essence, a traditional remedy in Southeast Asia. When a purified extract of the DKPs in chicken essence was administered to rats, it raised levels of serotonin, norepinephrine, and dopamine in the prefrontal cortex. This area of the brain is crucial to attention, planning, memory, learning and decision making, and serotonin is central to cognitive processing, mood, and sleep. Depressed rats which received oral doses of the extract escaped more quickly from a water maze. Other rats dosed with the DKPs improved their accuracy in a radial maze test. These results suggest that DKPs could provide therapeutic uses in the treatment of depression and in depression-induced cognitive impairments.

Interest in bioactive peptides found in foods has dramatically increased in recent decades. Research continues to uncover novel bioactive peptides and to reveal their possible functions and health benefits. A database, BIOPEP-UWM™, currently is collecting information about the biological activities of bioactive peptides, as well as documenting new peptide discoveries. Biopeptides which positively impact physiological processes could be useful in pharmaceuticals, and as food additives or functional foods.

"Functional foods" are foods which produce beneficial health effects. Some foods contain specific ingredients that produce these effects, while, as we have seen, other foods contain protein precursors which are broken down into biopeptides. Consumer awareness of these naturally-occurring, health-promoting products is growing rapidly. But how secure are the natural sources of these crucial biomolecules?

Natural Peptide Sources In Danger: Depleted Soils, Rising Co2, And Vanishing Nutrients

Natural sources of bioactive peptides are under threat from two directions. The soil in which food crops and livestock feed are grown is eroding and losing its vitamins and minerals. Global levels of carbon dioxide (CO2) are rising, resulting in damaging impacts on the nutritional content of cereals, fruits, and vegetables. These ecological developments potentially pose disastrous consequences for human health and the food security of two billion of the world's people.

Ninety-five percent of the world's food crops are grown in the uppermost layer of soil, the topsoil, which is typically less than a foot deep. This thin, precious layer of topsoil provides the vital nutrients plants require to grow and flourish. It takes 1000 years for one inch of topsoil to be created naturally. Yet around the world, topsoil is being eroded—washed away by rain and floods or blown away by the wind—partially because of intensive modern farming practices. The United Nations estimates that twenty-four billion tons of fertile soil are lost to degradation and erosion per year, affecting one third of the arable land in the world. Some experts estimate that only sixty years of topsoil is left.

Modern agriculture also strips nutrients from the soil and encourages other farming practices which result in less healthful foods. According to a 2004 study performed by scientists at the University of Texas at Austin, current crops of fruits and vegetables simply do not contain the same number of vitamins and minerals as they once did, even as recently as one hundred years ago. The researchers determined that from 1950 to 1999, forty-three different vegetables exhibited reductions in protein, vitamins B2 and C, iron, phosphorus, and calcium.

Lead researcher, Donald Davis, pointed to current farming practices as the primary culprit. "Efforts to breed new varieties of crops that provide greater yield, pest resistance and climate adaptability have allowed crops to grow bigger and more rapidly," he notes, "but their ability to manufacture or uptake nutrients has not kept pace with their rapid growth." (Scheer, 2011). Another study of twelve fresh vegetables demonstrated similar, significant declines in the levels of calcium, iron (down as much as 37%), potassium, Vitamin A, and Vitamin C (reduced 30%). One study concluded that the orange you eat today contains eight times less Vitamin A than an orange eaten by your grandparents. And if these threats to human nutrition and health were not already alarming enough, the rising levels of carbon dioxide on the planet also are severely affecting the nutritional quality of our food, including the proteins which are crucial to the creation of bioactive peptides.

Ninety-nine percent of our Earth's atmosphere is composed of two gases, nitrogen (78%) and oxygen (21%). The remaining one percent consists of several trace gases, including carbon dioxide (CO2). Levels of CO2 have risen and fallen dramatically over the life of the planet, but they have climbed rapidly since the beginning of the Industrial Revolution. It is believed that in the early decades of the twenty-first century, carbon dioxide levels were at their highest point matched only at a time that existed fourteen million years ago.

Plants require CO_2 to live and grow, but higher levels of this gas produce paradoxical effects on plant growth and nutritional composition. Elevated levels of CO_2 boost rates of photosynthesis in plants and raise their productivity and yields. However, those gains may come at the cost of nutritional quality. Scientists note that plants grow faster but they contain more starch, while amounts of protein, vitamins, and vital trace minerals decline. Animals which consume grasses and livestock feeds that contain less protein will provide less protein for human consumption.

Bees rely on flowers to supply pollen for the protein they need for their health and development. However, a study of a late autumn, North American flower called goldenrod demonstrated that elevated atmospheric carbon dioxide is reducing the amount of protein in the goldenrod's pollen. If similar declines in protein are occurring in other bee pollen sources, the lower nutritional quality could potentially impair the health and longevity of these crucial pollinators and cause serious environmental and economic consequences.

Scientists are particularly concerned about the impacts of rising levels of CO_2 on the nutritional value of rice, a crucial daily source of calories for over two billion people. Research indicates that different strains of rice grown in field conditions which simulate the levels of CO_2 expected by the end of this century exhibit significant, declines in protein, Fe (iron), and Zn (zinc). Reductions in the B-vitamins were as high as 30%. Comparable studies of other major food crops have demonstrated similar results. Wheat showed declines in protein, iron and zinc, and iron and zinc were reduced in soybeans and field peas. Maize (corn) and sorghum showed fewer effects. Experts believe that in the future, these nutritional deficiencies might significantly impact human health and food security, especially for the hundreds of millions of people who rely heavily on a single source of food, such as rice.

At the other end of the scale, however, is another paradoxical consequence of the loss of nutrients in our foods. According to an article in the Journal of the Academy of Nutrition and Dietetics, people may be consuming more starchy foods in greater quantities to compensate for the decline in their nutritional quality, contributing to the rising levels of obesity in many countries. One writer speculated that we are headed for a "bizarre world in which we are surrounded by food that we can't get enough of while, in reality, we're starving while simultaneously becoming obese." (Suglia, 2018). Rising levels of CO2 are diminishing the nutritional value and effectiveness of the foods we consume to provide bioactive peptides to our bodies.

We have learned that several foods, including milk, eggs, meat, and cereal crops, contain proteins composed of bioactive peptides. However, these peptides are encrypted, or inactive, until they are unlocked by digestion, fermentation, cooking, or other forms of food processing. After the peptides are liberated, they exert their effects directly in the stomach or intestines, or travel through the bloodstream and affect multiple body systems and physiological processes. Researchers have discovered that food-derived biopeptides have the capacity to lower blood pressure in hypertensive humans and rats, improve cognitive performance in depressed rats, prevent blood clots, and kill microbes, tumors, and cancer cells, among other beneficial health effects.

Unfortunately, just as more people are becoming interested in the life-enhancing and life-extending benefits of bioactive peptides, their natural sources are increasingly threatened by soil depletion and rising levels of carbon dioxide. How will people obtain these crucial biomolecules in the future? Peptide research performed by the Soviet Union during the Cold War in the 1980s began to provide the answer to this question.

Chapter Three

Russian Peptide Bioregulators and Anti-Aging Science

Interest in the field of peptide science has intensified rapidly in just the past decade or so. British physiologists William Bayliss and Ernest Starling made the first discovery of a bioactive peptide in 1902, when their experiments on dogs revealed the existence of secretin, a peptide hormone. Secretin is released by cells in the small intestine during digestion and stimulates effects in the stomach, pancreas, and small intestine. This research was particularly significant because it showed how chemical messengers in the body affected physiological processes. In 1922, therapeutic use of bioactive peptides began with the discovery of insulin as a life-saving treatment for diabetes. By the 1950s, researchers reported success using purified extracts of a polypeptide, adrenocorticotropic hormone (ACTH), from animal pituitary glands to treat disorders such as rheumatoid arthritis.

The systematic identification of gastrointestinal peptides by several scientists during the 1960s sparked the discovery of many new bioactive peptides. The pituitary gland is often called the "master gland" because the tiny organ controls most of the other hormone-secreting glands. In 1977, Roger Guillemin and Andrew Schally, former scientific colleagues turned bitter rivals, shared a Nobel Prize in Medicine with Rosalyn S. Yalow for their work on the peptide hormones that control pituitary hormone secretion. As researchers continued to study peptides in the following years, they began to recognize that gastrointestinal peptides also were expressed in the brain. Neuropeptides, crucial signaling molecules in the brain, now are central players in the science of neuroendocrinology.

Recent research is indicating that some of these biomolecules, such as NGF or Neuropeptide Y, not only play key roles in the regulation of hunger and metabolism, but also may be pivotal in the biological processes of aging. During the same period as the American Nobel winners' work on pituitary peptides, two Russian researchers, Vladimir Khavinson and Vladimir Anisimov, started investigating the treatment of aging with peptide extracts. Khavinson and Anisimov have been pursuing this research for nearly fifty years. Describing aging as the "the most intricate problem of medicine and biology," they have focused on repairing or reversing aging on a cellular level through the use of peptide extracts from several key glands, including the pineal gland and thymus gland. (Khavinson and Anisimov, 2009).

The pineal gland is located deep in the center of your brain and secretes melatonin, which regulates your circadian rhythms and certain reproductive hormones. The thymus gland is in your chest, behind your breastbone and between your lungs. It grows until you reach puberty, then begins to shrink and is replaced by fat. It produces the hormone thymosin, which stimulates the release of T-lymphocytes, white blood cells which fight bacterial and viral infections. These T-cells migrate to your lymph nodes and become part of your body's disease defense system for the rest of your life. Khavinson and his colleagues have produced extracts from the thymus gland that, they claim, boost the production of T-cells in aged animals and restore the function of their immune systems.

Back In The USSR: Vladimir Khavinson, Thymus Extracts, And Aging

During the late 1960s and early 1970s, in what was then the USSR, two Russian military medical students, Vladimir Khavinson and Vyacheslav Morozov, began extracting peptides from calf thymuses. As Khavinson, who currently calls himself a bio gerontologist, explained in a 2013 interview, "Our main idea was to affect the regulation of hypothalamus, pineal gland and thymus by using peptides. We tried to get these peptides from the corresponding organs, and we did not know at that time that A.V. Schally, and his colleagues, also worked on this, and he was awarded the Nobel Prize for this discovery in 1977." (Rattan, 2013). Although the interview often is unclear as to the dates of his activities, Khavinson and his colleague obtained laboratory space and began testing the thymus extracts on young mice exposed to radiation. They chose to start working with the thymus first, because its role in the immune system and the production of antibodies was well understood at the time.

But then the Russian researchers decided to use older mice because aging provides the "best pathology model." (Ibid). As Khavinson explained, "You take young and old animals, see their differences, and do your treatment and see if you can make the old mice healthier." (Ibid). Khavinson noted that older animals have weaker immune systems which manufacture fewer, feebler T-cells, but, he claimed, "Our extract from thymus stimulated the activity of T-lymphocytes, and the restoration of the immune function in old animals was very striking." (Ibid). He pointed out to the interviewer that the first drug developed from the thymus extract, called thymalin, was sold as a pharmaceutical product in Russia, and was used by millions of people with no side-effects.

Khavinson began collaborating with Vladimir Anisimov in 1970. They tested the tumor-suppressing effects of pineal gland extracts and other substances and found that the extracts from the pineal gland suppressed tumors by 82%. They then directed their efforts to the investigation of the effects of the extracts on lifespan and aging. According to Khavinson's account, Anisimov began experiments to determine the toxic effects of the thymus and pineal extracts but found that there were not any toxic effects at all. The pineal gland extracts extended the lifespan of mice by 20% to 30% and demonstrated powerful tumor-suppressing abilities.

In 1975, the Russian scientists obtained permission from the USSR Health Ministry to begin testing their extracts on human subjects. Khavinson acknowledged that this process was easy because the Soviet Union did not have strict regulations or ethical committees overseeing such research. They started testing in general public clinics at twenty locations in the USSR. Dr. Khavinson patented thymalin in the USSR in 1978, and later received a U.S. patent on the extract. Ultimately, he worked on ten different drugs, including extracts from the retina of the eye.

Khavinson advanced to the rank of colonel and became the head of a special Military Medical Academy laboratory on bioregulation in 1982. They worked on developing "drugs to increase resistance of the military people to hazardous factors, especially to atomic weapons." (Rattan, 2013). Soviet military leaders also were concerned about the impacts of constant, low-level radiation on the crews of nuclear-powered submarines and the troops who manned nuclear missile silos. Because the U.S. and the Soviet Union were still fighting the Cold War at the time, both sides worked on the development of laser weapons capable of blinding enemy soldiers. Khavinson and his colleagues tested their retinal extracts in animals and found that they partially restored the retinas in laser-damaged eyes. The USSR Ministry of Defense gave him an award for this work, but fortunately, the Cold War ended before these biopeptide therapies were tested under actual battlefield conditions.

Post-Soviet Peptide Science

After the collapse of the Soviet Union in 1992, Khavinson and his associates organized the Institute of Bioregulation and Gerontology and they began to study peptide extracts as solutions for "gerontology problems." (Ibid). Six drugs that he developed are sold without prescriptions in Russia and Ukraine. They are used to stimulate immune function, restore melatonin levels in older people, and restore brain function, among other benefits. While these peptide compounds are intended to address specific, serious health issues, Khavinson noted that because normal aging causes the body's functions to deteriorate slightly, even healthy people can take his "geroprotectors" to help maintain vigor and vitality. He claimed that he has been injecting himself with a compound composed of peptides from the pineal gland, thymus, brain, heart, blood vessels, and other organs for ten days every year. Khavinson explained that physically and mentally he felt at least twenty years younger than his chronological age of 66 (at the time of the interview in 2013), although he did admit to lower energy levels.

Khavinson believed that, "peptides become available in the stomach after proteins are cut into small pieces, and then they penetrate the cells and regulate DNA." (Ibid). In a 2009 article co-written with Anisimov, the Russian biogerontologists reviewed their thirty-five years of research on peptide regulation of aging. They concluded that the involution, or degeneration, of the major organs underlies the aging process, accompanied by decreased levels of protein synthesis in the cells of the body. However, therapeutic interventions using peptide extracts from the organs of young animals induced cellular protein synthesis and substantial recovery of the body's functions. Administration of the extracts to animals extended their life by 25% to 31%, up to the specific-species lifespan limit. In humans, treatment with the compounds markedly improved physiological functions and significantly reduced mortality in different age groups.

In a lengthy web page titled, "Peptide Regulation of Ageing," Khavinson explains his decades of investigation of peptide bioregulators to prevent, repair, and reverse the biological processes of aging. He claims that "the regulating role of small peptides had never been discussed in the concepts of gene control of protein synthesis in higher organisms before we started the research." (Khavinson, n.d.). He argues that the true human lifespan is 110 to 120 years, but several decades are shaved off the average life because of changes in the structure and expression of our genes due to stress, environmental factors, or radiation. However, he and his colleagues developed methods for extracting low-molecular peptides from the thymus and pineal gland which restore the functions of these glands and extend the lifespan of animals in many experiments. The positive results of these tests in animals, including monkeys, have encouraged the Russian researchers to perform successful tests of the immune-enhancing, life-extending peptide extracts in elderly and senile humans.

Khavinson has been the Director of the St. Petersburg Institute of Bioregulation and Gerontology since 1992 and was the President of the International Association of Gerontology and Geriatrics (European Region) from 2011 to 2015. He has continued to publish his research, but almost exclusively in Russian-language journals, so his work does not appear to be well-known in many Western scientific circles. Several of his most recent publications focus on his analysis and elucidation of the precise mechanisms of the cellular interactions between bioactive peptides and genes.

Interest in the therapeutic applications of bioactive peptides has increased dramatically in just the recent decade, and Khavinson's provocative, promising work on their immune-boosting, anti-aging, geroprotective potential may begin to gain more traction in the years ahead.

Currently, over 150 peptide pharmaceuticals are in active development, with numerous potential therapeutic applications. Bioactive peptides build muscle mass and strength, prevent age-related bone loss, improve wound healing ... what else can they do for us? Modern peptide science is just beginning to uncover the multifunctional benefits of these amazing biomolecules.

Chapter Four

Modern Bioactive Peptide Science

Building on the last 120 plus years of peptide science, modern research continues to document the numerous health benefits of these powerful biomolecules. These biomolecules build muscle mass, strength, prevent age-related bone loss, and improve the texture and elasticity of the skin. They stimulate the defense of wounds against infection and take a lead role in wound healing and repair. Bioactive peptides have shown the ability to prevent and reverse premature aging at the cellular level. Russian biogerontologist Vladimir Khavinson and his colleagues are not the only researchers investigating the anti-aging potential of a variety of bioactive peptides. Scientists in Europe and the USA are studying several different biological processes and bioactive peptide treatments for the diseases and disorders that occur with aging.

Peptides To Prevent And Reverse Premature Aging

Research teams are targeting senescent cells, which are old or worn-out cells in the body that are no longer capable of replicating and renewing themselves. They cause inflammation and damage to other cells and body tissues, but young people can clear them out efficiently. However, as we age, our immune systems become weaker and the senescent cells accumulate and cause dysfunctions in physiological processes, resulting in signs of aging such as wrinkled skin and hair loss. Peter L.J. de Keizer, a Dutch expert in molecular medicine, has reported promising results in mice from the administration of a cell-penetrating peptide that selectively targets worn-out, broken-down cells and clears the way for healthy, new tissues to develop. The peptide works only on senescent cells, not healthy ones, and instructs the harmful cells to self-destruct.

Aging mice who received the infusions of the cell-penetrating peptide soon regrew fur in bald spots. After several weeks, they showed higher levels of cardiovascular fitness than mice who did not receive the infusions. They also regained healthy kidney function within a month of beginning treatment. According to De Keizer, his team administered the peptide to the mice three times a week for ten months without any noticeable side effects. While it is not yet clear that the cell-penetrating peptide extends lifespan, De Keizer is optimistic about its safety profile and its therapeutic potential in humans. He explains that "The common thread I see for the future of anti-aging research is that there are three fronts in which we can improve: The prevention of cellular damage and senescence, safe therapeutic removal of senescent cells, to stimulate stem cells—no matter the strategy—to improve tissue regeneration once senescence is removed." (Cell Press, 2017). Multiple research teams are working on all of these fronts, and peptides produced in the mitochondria appear to be exciting new weapons in their anti-aging arsenals.

Mitochondria are structures inside all the cells of our bodies that produce energy from food. They are often called the "powerhouses" of the cells, but scientists are learning that they also manufacture peptides which are crucial to metabolism and aging. One of these mitochondrial peptides, called humanin, has been shown to combat age-related diseases. Researchers recently announced that for the first time, they also have evidence which indicates that higher levels of humanin in the body are linked with greater health and longer life. The children of centenarians, people who live to be 100 one hundred or more, are statistically more likely to also live exceptionally long lives, and in one study they also had higher, more sustained levels of humanin.

A 2018 study also discovered that lower levels of humanin in people related to accelerated cognitive aging. Injections of the peptide in mice demonstrated the ability to delay age-related cognitive decline, potentially opening a path to anti-aging therapeutic interventions in people. Researchers believe that humanin acts by reducing inflammation in the brain and throughout the body. Another recently discovered mitochondrial peptide, called SHLP 2, demonstrates strong anti-diabetic effects and may be able to reverse or protect against neurodegenerative disorders such as Alzheimer's disease. Other bioactive peptides are demonstrating promising result in the prevention of age-related loss of bone and muscle.

Peptides Prevent Age-Related Bone Loss

Over 40 million American men and women who are fifty years or older are threatened with age-related bone dysfunction, including low bone mass and osteoporosis. Osteoporosis causes the bones to become weak and brittle and more prone to fracture. It occurs when old bone cells die, but the growth of new bone cells fails to keep the same pace. Researchers have reported a link between senescent cells and bone loss in mice. Biologist Anja Nohe has shown that administering a peptide called CK2.3 in a mathematical model of a mouse increased bone mineral density. Unlike other current therapies for osteoporosis, this peptide is the only one that simultaneously increases the breakdown of old bone while stimulating the regrowth of new bone tissue.

Another potential therapy for age-related bone loss has been stirring a great deal of interest in recent years: collagen peptides. Numerous studies have demonstrated that bioactive collagen peptides produce a variety of beneficial health effects, including increased bone density in post-menopausal women. In a recent study, 131 post-menopausal women aged forty-six to eighty with age-related loss of bone mineral density were given a supplement containing either collagen peptides or a placebo for a year. Testing revealed that bone mineral density increased significantly in the women who received the collagen peptide supplement compared to the control group.

Peptides Fight Periodontal Disease And Loss Of Bone In The Jaw

Many people suffer from a dental disease called periodontitis, which causes inflammation of the gums and bone loss around the teeth. If untreated, teeth become loose and fall out or must be extracted, leading to a loss of bone in the jaw. Dentures only aggravate the bone loss. A protein called BMP-2 is known to stimulate the production of new bone cells, however high levels can cause inflammation and tumors. The peptide OP3-4 prevents bone decay and triggers the specialization of new bone cells. When OP3-4 is combined with BMP-2 and injected into mice jawbones, the compound stimulates an increase in bone mass around the site of the injection. The peptide-protein combination may offer new hope to people with tooth and bone loss.

Peptides Fight Age-Related Muscle Loss And Build Muscle Mass And Strength

As early as age forty, a condition called sarcopenia begins, which is where humans begin to lose muscle and the muscles that do exist weaken. Sarcopenia leads to a higher risk for falls and frailty. In a recent study, fifty-three men aged sixty-five or older with sarcopenia performed resistance training for three months. They then drank a supplement containing either collagen peptides, or a placebo, as soon as possible after the exercise session, but no later than an hour. At the end of the study, the men who took the supplement were leaner and stronger, with increased muscle mass, increased bone mass, and better motor control than those in the control group.

A similar study was performed in fifty-seven younger men who exercised or played sports for recreation. After twelve weeks of resistance training three times per week and the daily consumption of a collagen peptide supplement, those taking the supplement showed a significant increase in fat-free mass and demonstrated a slight increase in strength compared to the placebo group. The results of a comparable program of resistance training and collagen peptides for seventy-seven premenopausal women were even more promising. While all the women reduced their fat mass and increased their strength, the women who received the supplement lost more body fat, gained more fat free mass, and demonstrated greater hand-grip strength and leg strength than the women in the control group.

Could it even be possible to achieve similar results without physical exercise? A study of mice revealed that during exercise, muscles release a peptide, an "exercise factor" called musclin, which increases physical endurance and muscle performance. Mice that were bioengineered to lack musclin had lower exercise tolerance than wild mice. When the musclin-deficient mice received infusions of the peptide, they regained their normal exercise capacity in just a week. Wild mice that were infused with the peptide ran faster and longer on a treadmill than wild mice given a placebo. These intriguing results suggest potential therapeutic uses in people experiencing muscle loss and muscle weakness, especially older people, or those who have experienced muscle atrophy and debilitation due to injury or illness. What if humans could not only get stronger, but look younger, too? Several bioactive peptides currently used to reduce wrinkles, increase firmness and elasticity, and restore a more youthful skin have demonstrated very exciting results.

Collagen Peptides Stimulate Healthier, Younger-Looking Skin

Numerous recent studies have demonstrated that consumption of collagen peptide supplements offers anti-aging benefits. The bioactive peptides improve skin texture, elasticity, and firmness;

reduce wrinkles; and rejuvenate skin at the cellular level. A trial of a collagen peptide extracted from the skin of a fish, the Nile tilapia, and then orally administered to mice, revealed marked improvement in the appearance and structure of their skin. The peptide was highly digestible, safe, and showed strong antioxidant properties, which played a key role in the skin improvements. Comparable results have been achieved in other trials using animals, and recent investigations of the effects of the peptides in humans have been very promising. In a 2014 study, sixty-nine women aged thirty-five to fifty-five ingested either a collagen peptide supplement or a placebo daily for eight weeks. At the end of the trial, the women who received the supplement showed statistically significant improvement in skin elasticity compared to the control group.

A 2015 report examined clinical trials in Japan and France of specific collagen peptides from fish and pig sources. In the first study, sixty Japanese women, forty to fifty-nine years old, consumed either the peptide or a placebo for fifty-six days. In the second trial, forty white French women, aged forty to sixty-five, ingested either the peptide or a placebo for eighty-four days. In addition, skin from the thigh of a forty-nine-year-old woman was cultured in a laboratory and treated with the peptides. The researchers concluded that the pork peptide increased skin hydration by as much as 28% after eight weeks of treatment and significantly improved the collagen network in the skin.

A twelve-week clinical trial in 2018 of collagen peptides also reported promising results for sixty-four women who were forty to sixty years old with accelerated aging of the skin due to sun damage. After oral ingestion of 1000 mg of the supplement for six weeks, skin hydration was seven times greater in the test group than in the control group taking a placebo. Wrinkle improvement was ten times greater in the women who took the peptide. Their crow's feet and skin elasticity had significantly improved by six weeks. These are just a few of the many recent clinical trials of collagen peptides which are confirming that oral consumption of these biomolecules can deliver smoother, stronger, more hydrated skin in just a few weeks. Bioactive peptides can also help repair and heal skin and other body tissues that have been damaged by injury or disease.

Peptides Improve Wound Healing

Researchers have found that bioactive peptides derived from a wide variety of animal sources are capable of stimulating the repair and healing of wounds. In a recent European study, laboratory tests demonstrated that collagen peptides from pork promoted wound closure in both young and old connective tissue cells called fibroblasts.

Salamanders are small amphibians that can perform an amazing trick: they can regenerate damaged organs and regrow tails and limbs lost in fights with predators. This process begins with the closure of the wound by a layer of skin cells which happens very quickly in salamanders—less than ten hours—compared to the two to three days it takes for mammals.

According to a 2014 study, the secret to the salamanders impressive wound-healing ability may be a small peptide in their skin. This short peptide, tylotoin, consisting of only twelve amino acids, demonstrated the ability to stimulate epidermal growth factor (EGF) in a mice model of a deep wound in the skin. Eight days after the injury, the wounds in the tylotoin-treated mice were 65% smaller than the wounds of the control group. Tylotoin enhanced the development of new skin and connective cells and the formation of new blood vessels, accelerating wound closure and healing.

Ocean fish and other sea creatures are furnishing multiple new collagen peptides to treat cuts, burns, and other wounds. Chinese researchers performed Caesarian sections on pregnant rats and then administered peptides from marine fish at five-day intervals over the following fifteen days. The study reported stronger wound tissue and increased collagen and smooth muscle fiber formation at the incision site in the rats who received the infusion compared to the control group. A 2019 investigation of collagen peptides derived from jellyfish reported that mice wounds treated with the peptides "showed remarkable signs" of wound closure, tissue regeneration, and improved collagen formation. (Felician, 2019).

Researchers are investigating other collagen peptides from the same fish as "an effective and promising" treatment for severe burn wounds in people. (Hu, 2017). A 2020 study of collagen peptides from the skin of both the Nile tilapia and the Atlantic salmon revealed that the biomolecules performed several complex tasks when applied to wounds on rats. They decreased inflammation, stimulated the formation of collagen, and increased the growth of new blood vessels. The researchers also discovered one of the keys to the peptides' wound-healing powers. The collagen peptides upregulate an antimicrobial peptide which increased colonization of the wound by beneficial microbes and decreased colonization by harmful microflora. The rat wounds treated with the collagen peptides from both fish sources demonstrated significantly increased healing rates.

Wound healing is a complex process which requires the participation of several different types of cells. Researchers are discovering that antimicrobial peptides (AMPs), also called host defense peptides (HDPs), don't just directly combat harmful microbes such as bacteria, viruses, and fungi. These bioactive peptides also take lead roles in the coordination of the other biological activities involved in wound repair and healing.

Chapter Five

Host Defense Peptides and the Human Viral Shield

According to Russian folklore, soaking a frog in a pail of milk will prevent it from going sour. It turns out that the skin of the Russian brown frog produces a slime that is full of peptides that can destroy bacteria and other harmful microbes. These antimicrobial peptides (AMPs) are called Cationic Host Defense Peptides or Host Defense Peptides (HDPs). Russian scientists tested some of the peptides in the lab and found they were as effective against Salmonella and Staphylococcus bacteria as some prescription antibiotics. Researchers have discovered that a peptide in the slimy mucus on the skin of a South Indian frog kills the H1 flu virus. They named the antiviral peptide "urumin" after an ancient Indian sword. Unvaccinated mice that received a nasal formulation of urumin were protected against lethal doses of some influenza viruses. Studies of other antiviral frog peptides may yield promising therapies for viruses such as Zika, dengue fever, and SARS-Cov-2.

Some host defense peptides act directly to destroy harmful microbes including bacteria, viruses, fungi, and parasites. Scientists are discovering that they also take multiple, leading roles in many other physiological responses to wounds and infections. They modulate the immune system response to infection and possess wound healing and anti-inflammatory properties. They have anti-tumor and anti-cancer properties. Microbiologists increasingly stress the complex, multifunctional, interconnected activities, and effects of host defense peptides in the human body.

The Body Responds To Microbial Invaders: Innate And Adaptive Immunity

Harmful microorganisms in countless numbers exist in our natural environments, in the air, on surfaces, and in our food and water. Fortunately, our bodies are equipped with immune systems that have evolved many intricate, sophisticated, and powerful defenses against these microscopic enemies. The immune system is divided into two major types: adaptive or innate. Adaptive immunity occurs after a person has been exposed to an antigen from a pathogen, either through infection or vaccination. It can take days or weeks for the adaptive immune system to establish a response, but it is targeted for a specific pathogen. Adaptive immunity mobilizes T cells and B cells and antibodies to attack and destroy the microbial invaders. The adaptive immune system will remember the pathogen so that future invasions can be dealt with quickly and easily.

The innate immune system is roughly a billion years old and evolved as a basic defense against infection. Its response is a natural biological activity which does not depend upon previous infection or vaccination, as in adaptive immunity. Instead, the innate immune system reacts automatically to a pathogen through a complex series of activities designed to eliminate the threat or stimulate the adaptive immune system to craft a specific response to it. Innate immunity marshals a host of specialized cells such as neutrophils, mast cells, and macrophages that attack the pathogen and recruit other immune cells to the site of the infection. Antimicrobial peptides or host defense peptides (HDPs) are a vital part of innate immunity and link the innate and adaptive immune systems. Scientists are investigating the leading roles played by HDPs in stimulating, coordinating, and amplifying the body's defenses against microbial pathogens.

Host Defense Peptides: Defensins And Cathelicidins

Over five thousand host defense peptides (HDPs) have been identified to date. Because they are primarily found in tissues and organs that are vulnerable to airborne pathogens, such as the skin, nose, and lungs, they act as the first line of defense against bacteria, viruses, and other harmful microorganisms. They have been shown to eliminate the pathogen before the infection causes any symptoms. As mentioned in the introduction and chapter one, HDPs are divided into two main families based on their molecular structure: defensins and cathelicidins. Defensins are manufactured by leukocytes, or white blood cells, such as neutrophils and leukocytes, and by the epithelial cells that line the surfaces of our skin and organs. They typically are comprised of eighteen to forty-five amino acids. There are ten human defensins that are currently known. Although originally studied for their powerful antibacterial properties, defensins have demonstrated strong antiviral activities. They also function as signaling molecules to summon other immune cells to the site of the infection and regulate inflammation.

Cathelicidins are precursor proteins that release bioactive peptides with direct microbicidal activity against harmful microorganisms. The only human cathelicidin-derived HDP is called LL-37. It is produced by neutrophils and other immune cells such as mast cells and macrophages and is found in cells, fluids, tissues, and organs throughout the body. The peptide LL-37 demonstrates the ability to attack and destroy bacteria, viruses, and fungi. It also energizes a broad spectrum of responses to injuries and wounds, including regulation of inflammation, attracting immune cells to the site of the infection, and stimulating wound closure and healing.

Host Defense Peptides Battle Bacteria And Fungi

The antimicrobial activities of HDPs have been extensively investigated. Human skin furnishes one of the most crucial protective barriers against harmful organisms. Human skin produces sweat, which spreads antimicrobial substances over our skin, protecting the body from infections in scratches, cuts, and insect bites. One of these microbicidal substances in sweat is a powerful bioactive peptide called dermicidin. Dermicidin works by drilling channels in the cell membranes of microbial invaders, which results in the uncontrolled flow of water and ions into the bacterial cells, eventually causing their destruction. Dermicidin has demonstrated potency against bacteria such as Mycobacterium tuberculosis and Staphylococcus aureus. It is also effective against fungi.

HDPs derived from animals, insects, and amphibians exhibit powerful anti-fungal activity. Three defensins found in rabbits kill Candida albicans, and others are effective against the fungi that cause the disease called Valley Fever. Cecropins are peptides derived from the giant silk moth which kill disease-causing Aspergillis species and other fungi but are not harmful to mammalian cells. Frog skin has proven to be a rich source of antimicrobial peptides. Magainins are peptides produced in the skin of the African clawed frog that have shown the ability to inhibit the growth of C. albicans. A South American tree frog manufactures dermaseptins that are active against a broad range of fungi. Dermaseptins also kill protozoa, parasites, viruses, and bacteria in laboratory testing, and have exhibited anticancer and antimicrobial effects in rats and mice.

HDPs show great potential as treatments for several serious bacterial infections. Human defensins kill E. coli cells in less than thirty minutes in lab tests. LL-37 reduced the growth of the bacteria that causes the deadly disease, anthrax, by 50% in cell cultures. Human defensins protected mice injected with lethal doses of anthrax. HDPs from a variety of different species are under investigation for their possible use against bacteria which have become resistant to antibiotics, commonly called "superbugs." Methicillin-resistant Staphylococcus aureus (MRSA) has become a matter of increasing concern to public health officials because it cannot be treated successfully by most antibiotics, even some of those considered of last resort. Researchers are discovering potential new treatments for MRSA and other superbugs in bioactive peptides found in the tiny freshwater animal, the hydra; frog skin; and a recently identified biomolecule called 1018.

German researchers have discovered that the hydra produces an antimicrobial peptide, arminin 1a, that demonstrates powerful activity against a broad spectrum of bacteria, including MRSA. Researchers have identified ten HDPs in skin secretions from the African clawed frog which are effective against S. aureus and E. coli. Two of the HDPs exhibited potent activity against MRSA skin infections. Another antibiotic-resistant bacterium, Pseudomonas aeruginosa, causes severe, often fatal infections in burn wounds and in the eye, ear, and lung. In 2010, researchers in Italy reported that several antimicrobial peptides derived from frog skin increased the survival rate of worms infected with P. aeruginosa.

A Canadian research team identified a peptide they named IDR-1018 (Innate Defense Regulator) with powerful abilities to destroy and prevent the biofilms that help protect drug-resistant bacteria from antibiotics. In lab tests, IDR-1018 blocked a bacterial chemical signal crucial to biofilm development in less than thirty minutes, potentially opening a new path to the treatment of stubborn drug-resistant pathogens. The bacterium that causes tuberculosis is notoriously resistant to antibiotics and is commonly treated with a combination of drugs over several months. Researchers tested IDR-1018 and two related peptides, IDR-1002 and IDR-HH2, on mice infected with Mycobacterium tuberculosis for two months, in a model of long-term pulmonary tuberculosis in humans.

The mice received infusions of the peptides in their lungs three times per week. After fifteen days and thirty days of treatment, administration of 1018 and HH2 produced "a very strong and significant reduction in bacteria." (Rivas-Santiago, 2013).

Microscopic examination of the lung tissue in the mice treated with the peptides revealed that significantly less of the lung area was affected by pneumonia than in the control group. Interestingly, the scientists do not attribute these results to the direct antimicrobial activities of the peptides. They suggest that the IDRs have complex and multifunctional effects on the immune system at the cellular level that stimulate the recruitment of innate immune cells to fight the bacteria, suppress excessive inflammation, and amplify the adaptive response.

Host Defense Peptides, Viruses, And The Viral Shield

Researchers have established the virucidal properties of HDPs against a wide range of viruses in cell cultures. Defensins and cathelicins exhibit the ability to inhibit the infectivity and reduce the replication of viruses, including influenza, zika, rhinovirus, herpes simplex virus, and HIV. In lab tests, defensins have demonstrated strong activity against adenoviruses that cause infections of the lower respiratory tract, stomach and intestine, bladder, skin, and eyes. These infections are typically mild, but they can become serious, even fatal, in immune-compromised people. Defensins added to cell cultures of adenovirus reduced its growth by 96% and at higher doses halted the viral activity completely.

Peptides from many different species are under investigation for antiviral activity. Frog skin secretions, valuable for their antibacterial and antifungal properties, also furnish HDPs with potent antiviral effects. Investigators tested fifteen peptides from a variety of frog species and discovered that several of them inhibited HIV infection of T cells without damaging the T cells. Plant peptides called cyclotides have demonstrated virucidal effects against influenza, dengue fever, and HIV. A bioactive peptide isolated from scorpion venom, mucroporin, demonstrated antiviral effects against measles, flu viruses, and SARS-CoV in cell cultures and inhibited Hepatitis B infection in mice. A 2020 study successfully tested a peptide derived from the cowpox virus protein CPXV012 against a wide range of enveloped viruses, including herpes simplex virus-1, hepatitis B virus, HIV-1, and Rift Valley fever virus.

Because several bioactive peptides are active against multiple unrelated enveloped viruses, scientists theorize that these biomolecules all possess a common trait, called *interfacial activity.* The researchers tested their hypothesis by selecting several interfacially-active peptides without known antiviral activity and tested them on several viruses, including influenza, dengue, herpes simplex, and human adenovirus. The peptides powerfully suppressed the growth of all enveloped viruses tested at low concentrations which are safe for human cells. These and other bioactive peptides, which exhibit broad spectrum antiviral activity, are promising candidates for new antiviral drugs.

New antiviral compounds are especially crucial given the current global pandemic of the novel coronavirus, SARS-CoV-2. According to a recent study, computer modeling suggests that a peptide derived from a frog, dermaseptin-S9, can prevent the attachment of the SARS-CoV-2 spike protein to the surface of the ACE-2 receptor in human cells. Investigators recently reported that a peptide isolated from a mouse defensin, P9R, exhibited virucidal activities against the enveloped SARS-CoV-2, MERS-CoV, SARS-CoV, 2009 swine flu virus, bird flu virus, and a non-enveloped rhinovirus. An in vivo study showed that P9R protected mice against a lethal dose of the 2009 swine flu virus, which is an enveloped virus like the coronavirus. Many researchers are investigating the potential anti-Covid-19 activity of another antimicrobial peptide found in human breast milk, lactoferrin (LF). This biomolecule has demonstrated antiviral activity against a wide range of viruses, including SARS-CoV, because it suppresses their ability to replicate.

Lactoferrin (LF) does not just combat the virus after infection, it has also been shown to boost the body's ability to prevent viral infections by stopping the entry of viruses into cells, either through blocking cellular receptors, or directly binding to the virions. LF is one of the primary compounds in the mucosal secretions of tissues and organs that are directly exposed to pathogens. Examples of these tissues and organs include the nose, lungs, and gastrointestinal tract, making LF a crucial part of the first line of defense against microbial invaders, including viruses. As one study suggested, "These antiviral mechanisms highlight the possibility that baseline expression of CDHP could create an 'antiviral shield' at mucosal surfaces and prevent replication and spread of the virus if upregulated after initial infection." (Mookherjee, 2020). Researchers believe that LF is a strong candidate for upregulation in mucosa through formulations administered as a nasal spray or taken orally. If patients are treated with these therapies soon after becoming sick with the flu, COVID-19, or another virus, the LF formula could stop the virus in its tracks and significantly shorten the recovery time.

Host Defense Peptides Destroy Tumors And Cancer Cells

More than 170 bioactive peptides, including HDPs like magainins, cecropins, and defensins, have demonstrated anticancer properties. In lab tests, a peptide fragment derived from lactoferricin B, an antimicrobial peptide in cow's milk, killed stomach cancer cells within twenty-four hours. Scientists injected a small peptide, angiotensin-(1-7), into mice that were growing human lung cancer tumors and a saline solution into a control group, every day for six weeks. At the end of the trial, the weight of the tumors treated with the peptide had decreased by about 60%, while the tumors in the saline-treated group had grown larger. The peptide inhibits angiogenesis, or the growth of blood vessels that supply nutrients to the tumors. The researchers previously have reported promising results in using angiotensin-(1-7) to treat breast, colon and brain tumors. Anticancer peptides may furnish relatively low-cost treatments without the harsh side effects of radiation and chemotherapy.

A research team has discovered that when therapy-sensitive cancer cells die, they release a peptide, PAF, with the ability to kill the therapy-resistant cancer cells. It also reduced the growth of metastatic tumors in mice. The newly discovered "killer peptide" is especially promising as a safe therapeutic agent because it acts only on cancer cells and spares healthy tissue. A study performed in 2016 demonstrated that psaptides, small peptides consisting of five amino acids derived from a human protein called prosaposin, caused metastatic tumors to shrink significantly in a mice model of ovarian cancer. Psaptide can trigger powerful anti-angiogenic and anti-inflammatory effects and could potentially inhibit the spread of breast, prostate, and lung cancer.

Host Defense Peptides Modulate The Immunse System Response To Infection

Although originally known for their antimicrobial properties, in recent years researchers have discovered that HDPs are "immunomodulatory," meaning they directly impact and influence the immune system. HDPs play complex and multifunctional roles in the body's innate and adaptive immune systems' response to disease and injuries. Some defensins and the cathelicidin LL-37 are chemotactic, attracting various types of immune cells to the site of an infection or wound. Other defensins influence the development and specialization of the immune cells and galvanize adaptive immunity through stimulating the migration of T cells.

Some HDPs regulate the suppression of chemicals called cytokines which stimulate pro-inflammatory responses, preventing excessive and harmful inflammation. LL-37 has been shown to block several inflammatory responses and to limit the damage caused by bacterial products. For example, an endotoxin is a poisonous lipopolysaccharide (LPS) produced by certain bacteria and released when the bacterial cell disintegrates, causing fever, severe diarrhea, and shock. LL-37 partially protected mice against lethal endotoxic shock after they were injected with LPS. Mice that were injected with E. coli LPS all died within four to six hours. However, when the mice were given an injection of LL-37 fifteen minutes after receiving the LPS, half of the animals survived. Some scientists argue that although HDPs can directly suppress microbial growth and spread, their most important function is to modulate the immune system. They mobilize immune cells such as macrophages while limiting harmful inflammation. They also play key roles in the repair and healing of wounds.

Host Defense Peptides Are Crucial To Wound Healing

HDPs promote the healing of wounds through several different mechanisms. They stimulate the closure of the wound by new skin cells and induce the formation of new blood vessels. The new blood vessels bring oxygen and nutrients to the healing wound. Human β -defensins (HBDs) stimulate the migration and growth of skin cells, which may promote healing of skin wounds. Levels of HBDs increase in acute and chronic wounds, but the peptide is undetectable in healthy skin.

The multifunctional cathelicidin, LL-37, plays a crucial role in wound healing. Injury or inflammation triggers an increase in LL-37 in skin cells and white blood cells. Levels of LL-37 rise in the skin after it is cut and return to baseline after the wound has closed. One reason that microbiologists believe that LL-37 is a major player in the healing of new wounds is because lower levels of the peptide are found in chronic wounds, indicating that the deficiency may be causing the failure of the wound to heal. This theory is supported by experiments in mice which show that LL-37 has powerful wound-healing properties. The peptide acts as a growth factor for epithelial cells and stimulates the migration of skin cells. Host defense peptides are efficient multitaskers. They stimulate wound-healing, damp down excessive inflammation, and act directly against harmful microorganisms, while promoting the growth of beneficial microbes.

Host Defense Peptides Support Healthy Microflora In The Body To Maintain Homeostasis And Health

The antimicrobial activity of host defense peptides (HDPs) is well established. However, new research is focusing on how HDPs help to shape microbial communities within the host to promote a healthy microbiome, instead of solely acting to kill pathogens. Many different types of microflora live on and in the body, coexisting harmlessly with each other. In fact, microbiologists now believe that diverse commensal populations are crucial to physiological homeostasis and defense against disease. The wide variety of natural HDPs in many animals could result from "species-specific HDPs that have co-evolved to select specific microbial communities beneficial to that specific host, while possibly limiting other species." (Haney, 2019). Experiments with mice demonstrate that human defensins help maintain homeostasis in the gut. Treatment of diabetic rats with human LL-37 altered the gut microbiota toward a configuration common in diabetes-resistant mice. HPDs utilize various mechanisms to manage the microbial balance in your body, which maintains homeostasis and health.

Microbiologists still are unraveling all the mysteries of the complex, multifunctional, synergistic activities of host defense peptides (HDPs). They are major players in the innate immune system's response to infection and injury and activate adaptive immunity. They can degrade and destroy harmful microbes and maintain and manage communities of beneficial microflora on and in the body. They suppress excessive inflammation and participate in wound healing. Researchers are discovering that the role of host defense peptides (HDPs) goes well beyond their antimicrobial properties. These remarkable biomolecules seem to be more deeply implicated in physiological processes that build up and strengthen the body's health and homeostasis instead of only biological activities that break down and destroy.

The body is under constant, relentless attack from harmful bacteria and viruses, yet they rarely succeed in gaining entrance and starting an infection. This is because the cells that form the outer surface of the skin and the respiratory, gastrointestinal, and urogenital tracts present a physical barrier against pathogens and produce antimicrobial substances, including bioactive peptides. Some scientists suggest that increasing the production of host defense peptides (HDPs) such as lactoferrin in the mucosa and epithelial cells could help erect a "viral shield" to protect your bodies against diseases like the flu and the novel coronavirus, SARS-CoV-2.

Modern peptide science provides substantial evidence that enhancing and strengthening the body's unique collection of bioactive peptides produces powerful health benefits. But how can that work? Where can the body find a complete, convenient source of these crucial biomolecules?

Fortunately, Genostim Performance Labs has taken the lead in providing the solution. The next chapter explains how the HDPs and other key bio-active peptides in our Hexatide™ peptide extract renews and amplifies the vital components of your own peptidome, fortifies the body's viral shield, and rejuvenates the body at the cellular and even molecular level.

Chapter Six

The Genostim® Hexatide™: Bioactive Peptides for Health and Life

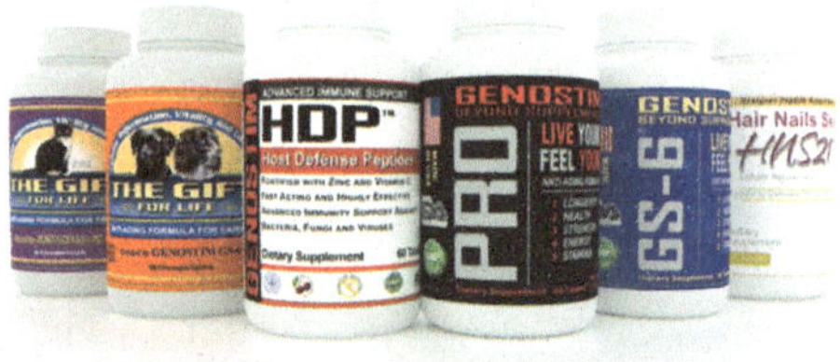

Peptides are made from amino acids which are literally the building blocks of the body. They naturally occur in raw foods however, eating these foods does not always guarantee that the correct number of amino acids were consumed, nor that the foods consumed were grown in nutrient-rich soils and have the proper bio-nutrients.

So how can one locate a complete and convenient source of these important bioregulators?

Enter Genostim®'s exclusive Hexatide™ peptide that is utilized in all Genostim® and The Gift For Life® products. Founded in 2006 by Lauriston Crockett III, Genostim® Performance Labs is the leader in peptide technologies and is dedicated to all-natural peptide formulas promoting cellular rejuvenation, health, and longevity in both humans and pets.

The Genostim® branded line of supplements contain the revolutionary Hexatide™ peptide complex with eighteen amino acids and twenty-one naturally occurring growth factors. These biomolecules aid the endocrine system, helping to regulate hormone activity and bring balance to the hypothalamic—pituitary—adrenal axis. More importantly now than ever before, the Genostim® Hexatide™ provides the body with a Viral Shield to boost the immune system utilizing cationic host defense peptides, or HDPs. These natural, biopeptide supplements are fast-acting and highly effective on the cellular level. Those who take Genostim® Products on a daily basis have reported receiving one or more of the following benefits: improved memory, calmer disposition/reduced physical and mental stress, accelerated healing, slowed aging process with joint pain relief, and increased sexual function.

The peptides in the Genostim® extract transmit chemical messages that affect many essential biological activities in the body. They exert anti-oxidative and anti-inflammatory effects which help regulate the hormone activity in the body's endocrine system and bring balance to the hypothalamic—pituitary—adrenal axis (HPA). The included naturally occurring growth factors and HDPs amplify the body's defenses against bacteria, viruses and fungi and synergistically modulate the immune system response to infection and injury, boosting cellular recovery and rejuvenation.

THE GENOSTIM® FORMULA: THE REVOLUTIONARY HEXATIDE™

The Genostim® and Gift For Life® supplement lines are embryonic peptide products. They are formulated from the highest quality, naturally occurring sources, primarily chicken embryo extracts. These embryo extracts are vital components of the Genostim® Hexatide™ formula. They powerfully boost the production of muscle cells, blood cells, and nerve cells. Embryonic extracts in conjunction with a nutrient mixture have been linked with promoting the production of bone tissue stem cells in elderly rats, potentially slowing aging. The extracts furnish biologically rich and all-natural sources of crucial peptides that interact with and regulate the endocrine system, including growth factors.

The revolutionary Hexatide™ peptide, a cutting-edge oligopeptide matrix, is designed to help the body signal its endocrine system to work in total homeostasis and at youthful levels. The endocrine system is the life force of the body. Without this Genostim® formula, the body could age poorly due to a toxic environment, poor food qualities, daily stress and finally our own DNA signaling. Genostim® utilizes a powerful, pharmaceutically standardized Hexatide™ that contains naturally occurring growth factors. These growth factors are made of clusters of low-molecular weight which, by their very nature, are quickly and easily assimilated and transported to their specific receptor sites.

The Naturally Occurring Growth Factors Found In Genostim® Products

Over twenty bioactive peptides called growth factors are found in Genostim® products. Each of these growth factors has unique, bio-stimulating properties: TGF-B (Transforming Growth Factor-Beta) peptides promote healing of wounds and are anti-inflammatory; TNF-A, TNF-B (Tumor Necrosis Factors Alpha and Beta) are peptides that increase cellular responsiveness to growth factors and induce signaling pathways that leads to cellular proliferation; CTGF (Connective Tissue Growth Factors) promote collagen accumulation in the body; EGF (Epidermal Growth Factors) are polypeptides that promote skin tissue growth and development, and speed the healing of wounds; NGF (Nerve Growth Factors) promote neural cell survival; FGF (Fibroblast Growth Factors) are essential to the development of the skeletal and nervous systems; IGF-1, IGF-2 (Insulin-like Growth Factors-1, 2) comprise a family of peptides that plays an important role in growth and development, and mediates many of the growth-promoting effects essential to liver, kidney and brain functions; GHK-Cu, or copper peptide, is a multifunctional compound with antioxidant and anti-inflammatory effects. GHK-Cu, attracts immune cells and activates wound healing through the stimulation of collagen and glycosaminoglycan synthesis in skin fibroblasts and promotes blood vessel growth.

Initial Clinical Trial

Genostim® Hexatide™ formula induces a highly significant increase in key adrenal hormones like 17-ketosteroid sulfates and 17-hydroxycorticosteroids. It has also been shown to increase plasma concentrations of DHEA, DHEA-S, and testosterone, all while normalizing elevated cortisol levels. Twenty-eight healthy male football players (age twenty to thirty-two) volunteered to participate in a twenty-one-day clinical trial. Blood was drawn and hormone levels measured before the start of the trial to establish a baseline for each of the players. After twenty-one days of consuming 200mg of Hexatide™ per day, with no modifications made to their diet or training, hormone levels were again measured in the Football players. The results confirmed that Hexatide™ significantly increased key anabolic hormones while improving recovery by reducing oxidative stress.

Few supplements can claim to have such a dramatic effect on testosterone levels and can legitimately claim to simultaneously boost these key anabolic hormones while reducing oxidative stress and delivering these benefits via a 100% natural and safe medium. No adverse effects have ever been observed or reported from using Genostim® or The Gift For Life® formulas. The only reported side effects include increased sex-drive, improved sleep & mood, and increased fat loss with lean muscle mass increased.

Genostim® Hexatide™ Peptides: Architects Of Health

It appears that Genostim® Performance Labs may already have developed what was called the preparation of the future by Eric Drexler, the pioneer of nano medicine. Genostim®'s Hexatide peptides are completely free of adverse side effects and they enhance the genetic abilities of the patient's organism. Rather than just fill in for the functions of damaged tissues, they help the body activate its own reserves supplied by nature. By and large, just two types of molecules maintain life: proteins, or peptides, that carry the information, and the DNA that also encodes specific information. The DNA is just a matrix because the molecule by itself performs no function. Only when a relevant peptide connects with a corresponding segment of the DNA will it trigger the synthesis of specific proteins, and this is the key to life.

The human body consists of one hundred trillion cells, and each of these cells is comprised of hundreds of millions of protein molecules. Proteins, or peptides, can be said to be the construction material of the body. They also function as true nano machines ~50-100 nm wide. Each of the hundreds of thousands of various proteins is distinguished by a unique structure, and every single protein has a specific task it performs within the body. Proteins can be broken down by digestion and other processes into bioactive peptides, which consist of small chains of amino acids, the building blocks of all life.

Because peptides are smaller than proteins and are already partially broken down, they may be more easily absorbed by the skin and digestive system. Chains of between three and six amino acids are called short-chain peptides, or bioregulators. The lower the molecular weight of a peptide, the more likely it is to be absorbed by the cells of the small intestine and exert its biological effects. Bioactive peptides exert direct and crucial effects on your body's physiological processes. The Genostim® Hexatide™ peptide complex includes amino acids and growth factors with anti-oxidative and anti-inflammatory effects, which enhance healthy longevity.

Genostim®'s Powerful Anti-Aging Effects

The maximum human life span is one hundred and ten years, based on the dates of birth and death of the longest-living persons that have been verified according to modern standards. However, the average lifespan remains seventy to seventy-five years throughout different countries, and this is believed to be the effect of premature aging syndrome. Humans have a capacity to live for another thirty to forty-five years. The modern era, with its sedentary lifestyle, excessive consumption of highly sugared, caffeinated energy drinks, and heavy reliance on synthetic vitamin supplements has generated a premature aging affect. All these cases shared the same symptoms of severe impairments of body systems which are critical to life: the immune, endocrine, nervous, cardiovascular, and reproductive systems.

Genostim® Performance Labs has dedicated over twenty years of research and development to find a solution that would lead to the complete recovery and increase human and animal longevity. We study how mechanisms of aging are developing and look for ways we can hold them back with the help of bioactive peptides. Through the continued development of our Genostim® and The Gift For Life® peptide products, we are able to introduce new technologies and help explain how some peptides can assist in antiaging; in other words, how they can protect and improve our long-term health without drugs and side effects.

The Genostim® Hexatide™ reduces mortality rates with its bioregulation technologies. This exclusive protein peptide is life changing and there are no drugs that can compare to this highly effective peptide with natural growth factors. Clinical research revealed that the Hexatide™ helps the body increase normal testosterone production in men and women, leading to an increase in libido, higher sperm count in men, delay of menopause in women, and slows the aging process in both sexes. Genostim®'s pet division, The Gift For Life®, has been administered to mature animals for over twenty years and increased their actual lifespan by 29% to 31%.

Genostim®'s Science: How It Works

The Genostim® Hexatide™ peptide extract has two primary mechanisms of action: First, it regulates the adrenal cortex hormone activity (androgens, glucocorticoids, mineral-corticoids). Second, it exerts cell-stimulating, cell-protective, and anti-oxidative properties at the cellular and tissue levels. The Hexatide™ (essential amino and short amino acid chains) assists the body in normalizing numerous cellular processes by activating the fibroblast growth factor receptors. When this occurs, healing is accelerated, and a variety of cellular processes are normalized/ stabilized. This cell-stimulating also helps the division of mature cells and significantly helps to decrease the mortality of older cells.

At the heart of Genostim®'s science is the endocrine system, a diverse collection of seven glands that secrete hormones. Genostim® acts to restore equilibrium to the hypothalamus-pituitary-adrenal axis (HPA), which helps the entire endocrine system achieve homeostasis and peak efficiency. The improved endocrine performance normalizes the secretion of crucial hormones, including bioactive peptides, which transmit signals between cells. Optimizing the cellular communication network boosts cellular growth, repair, and recovery, which enhances health and longevity and renews youthful vigor and vitality.

The Genostim® extract is complex. It is an embryonic peptide product and contains naturally occurring peptides derived from biologically rich sources like embryonic extracts including growth factors (not to be confused with growth hormones). It passes intact through the gut into the blood stream and is absorbed by the body primarily through a process called pinocytosis. Pinocytosis comes from the Greek for "cell drinking" and it enables a cell to ingest liquid droplets. Genostim® is characterized as an adaptogenic, meaning that it acts to modify and maintain the equilibrium of hormones secreted by the adrenal cortex. This adaptogenic activity is a consequence of the fine-tuning exerted on the adrenal cortex by the natural growth factors from the Hexatide™ peptide. The growth factors from the Hexatide™ peptides regulate adrenal cortex activity through paracrine signaling, and delivered chemical messages to nearby cells, which alter and restore the homeostasis of all the hormones secreted by the adrenal glands, as proven by the increase of urinary 17-KS-S.

These hormones are responsible for healing the parts of the human body that have been exposed to cellular stress. Genostim®'s exclusive Hexatide™

advanced peptide formula contains more than twenty naturally occurring bioregulators that support accelerated healing, thereby stabilizing cellular processes at a more youthful level. Cellular recovery and rejuvenation are the answers to a longer, healthier life.

Genostim® Renews And Strengthens The Body

When the immune system functions properly, it protects the body against any "invaders" that might negatively affect it, such as bacteria, viruses, or other pathogens. Genostim® Performance Labs' have been researching and producing all-natural peptide formulas which promote cellular rejuvenation and defense against bacteria and disease for over fourteen years. Our highest priority is to promote wellness through natural peptide products and to continue to research and share data on peptides' vital role as a Viral Shield in the body. Genostim® offers health protection and supports the 'antiviral shield' by assisting the immune system through enhancement of cell-to-cell communication and signaling immune cells for their vital functions, anti-oxidative (free radical scavenging) and anti-inflammatory actions.

Genostim® supports a six-fold increase in cation free radical scavenging and a seven-fold increase in anion free radical scavenging when compared to glutathione, one of the most potent anti-oxidative compounds known. Genostim®

demonstrates an eleven-fold increase in hydroxyl ions free radical scavenging when compared to L-Ascorbic acid (Vitamin C). These profound benefits maintain a balanced mitochondrial energy transfer (the underpinning of most chronic human conditions) with mitigation of inflammation and progression to ailments. These highly specialized bioactive peptides increase optimal homeostasis in the human HPA endocrine system supporting advanced HDP production. This is crucial for a peptide "antiviral shield." Genostim®'s ability to support and strengthen the body's defenses against dangerous microbes is particularly important given the emergence of the novel coronavirus, SARS-CoV-2, which began to sweep across the world in January 2020.

As we learned in the previous chapter, host defense peptides (HDPs), also known as antimicrobial peptides, have demonstrated the ability to destroy enveloped viruses like SARS-CoV-2, the virus that causes COVID-19. They damage the viral envelope, reducing the virions' infectivity, and limiting their ability to replicate. Antiviral peptides which are naturally present in human mucosal and epithelial cells, such as lactoferrin (LT), could be increased in these cells and tissues to create an "antiviral shield" that helps prevent the spread of the infection if upregulated soon after the initial infection with the coronavirus.

Genostim®'s Life-Enhancing, Life-Extending Benefits

Someone taking Genostim® products enjoys better sleep, more energy, increased muscle mass and density development, faster healing from injury and a boost to the Viral Shield. While Genostim® and The Gift For Life® products are not drugs and the statements presented here have not been evaluated by the Food and Drug Administration, nor is Genostim® or The Gift For Life® intended or claimed to diagnose, treat, cure, or prevent disease, it has been shown in clinical and medical applications to help:

- Raise testosterone
- Reduce cortisol
- Reduce oxidative stress/speed recovery/amazing joint pain relief
- Increase Androstenedione, DHEA-S, DHEA
- Raise adrenal hormone levels
- Decrease catabolism in cirrhosis patients
- Increase sexual drive
- Improve sleep
- Normalize insulin levels

Decades of research have confirmed that bioactive peptides found in our diet can exert profound effects upon cells, tissues, glands, organs, and even our entire bodies. Since most of our food sources are being grown in nutrient-depleted soil, we lack the needed bio-nutrients for our health. The naturally occurring bioactive peptides found in the Genostim® extract shows the potential to restore and recalibrate your immune system and to rejuvenate your body at the cellular and even molecular level. Genostim®'s revolutionary Hexatide™ peptide complex addresses the health problems caused by the modern sedentary lifestyle and excess dietary sugar by providing anti-inflammatory, anti-oxidative, anti-aging benefits.

The free radical's theory of aging is now generally accepted as the primary cause of deterioration in the human body. Oxygen from unstable molecular particles, known as free radicals, attaches to other molecules and damage healthy tissue. The body needs antioxidants to prevent or slow the breakdown of tissue by oxygen. Clinical studies conducted on patients aged fifty and over revealed the Hexatide™ treated group showed a 72% increase in disease-fighting antioxidants.

Physician-Tested

The Genostim® Hexatide™ peptides unique properties have amazed even those in the medical community. Our clinical tests not only confirmed many individual use cases and observations, but also revealed some key findings. This resulted in a more comprehensive clinical study that has been initiated to measure the potential benefit of the Genostim® Hexatide™ formula on elevated insulin and cholesterol levels.

Biopeptide science is advancing at a rapid pace, with a burst of scholarly interest in recent years. The antiviral properties of host defense peptides are generating renewed interest in the current environment of a global coronavirus pandemic and constant emergence of new pathogenic threats. Genostim® Performance Labs' highest priority is to promote wellness through natural peptide products and to continue to research and share data on peptides' vital role as a Viral Shield in the body. Genostim® Performance Labs is expected to be at the forefront of the cutting-edge developments in the field. What is the exciting future of the medical use of these remarkable biomolecules?

Chapter Seven

Recent Research and Future of Medical Use of Bioactive Peptides

Scientific research into the many potential therapeutic uses of bioactive peptides has intensified in recent years, with teams around the world investigating the complex, multifunctional, synergistic activities of these remarkable biomolecules. Some of the most recent studies have focused on their antimicrobial, anti-diabetic, anti-cancer, and anti-aging activities.

Next Generation Of Antimicrobial Drugs

Bioactive peptides are promising candidates for new antimicrobial drugs because they can destroy a broad spectrum of pathogens; work synergistically with many antibiotics; and have immunomodulatory effects. Currently just a few antimicrobial peptides (AMPs) are approved for clinical use with several more in advanced clinical trials. One human defensin has been shown to be a safe and effective treatment for nail fungal infections, which disappear after just a month of daily applications. The human cathelicidin, LL-37, is under investigation as a treatment for chronic infections of the middle ear. Histatin 3 is a peptide with twelve amino acids derived from the natural histatin found in human saliva. It is used as an oral rinse to treat infections of C. albicans, also called thrush.

Many researchers are focusing on the antiviral potential of AMPs or host defense peptides (HDPs) as an agent against the novel coronavirus, SARS-CoV-2, that has caused a global pandemic that has killed almost two million people as of January 2021. In June 2020, researchers reported the results of work that could contribute to the development of a peptide-based vaccine against the virus.

Anti-Cancer Activities Of Bioactive Peptides

Many research teams are investigating the potential of antimicrobial peptides (AMPs) or host defense peptides as an effective, less toxic cancer-fighting agents, called anti-cancer peptides (ACPs). AMPs are short peptides with a positive charge that disrupt the negatively charged cell membrane of many microbes, causing them to leak, rupture, and die. Some AMPs have shown the ability to target human tumor cells through the same mechanisms. Cancer cell membranes have higher net negative charges than normal cells due to a few factors, increasing their susceptibility to destructive AMP interactions. Other features of the cancer cells may increase their attraction for AMPs and promote cytotoxic activity. In lab tests, the human cathelicidin, LL-37, disrupts cancer cell membranes by opening a hole in the membrane that allows it to penetrate the cell and block essential cellular processes, resulting in cell death. The activity of LL-37 against melanoma is currently being investigated in a clinical trial.

The venom of spiders and hornets provides cancer-fighting peptides, according to recent studies. A peptide called gomesin, extracted from a Brazilian spider, shows anti-cancer activity against mouse and human leukemia and melanoma cells. Mastoparan-C (MP-C), a peptide isolated from the venom of the European hornet, showed anti-cancer activity against non-small cell lung cancer, prostate cancer, and human breast cancer cell lines. Other peptides, such as cecropin from the silkworm and Magainin 2 from the African clawed frog, demonstrate anti-cancer activities without damaging normal human or mouse cells. Several peptides derived from various frogs have shown significant activities against cancer cells, including large cell lung cancer, breast cancer, melanoma, and prostate cancer. Marine sources, such as fish, crabs, and sea squirts, provide AMPs that have also demonstrated potent anti-cancer activities.

These anti-cancer peptides are especially promising because they are effective at low concentrations and are non-toxic to normal human cells. They may help overcome the problem of cancer cells becoming resistant to treatment by many of the drugs currently used in chemotherapy, called multi-drug resistance (MDR). Other AMPs are effective against tumor growth because they inhibit angiogenesis, or the development of blood vessels that bring nutrients to the tumor. However, certain limitations in the clinical use of ACPs still need to be overcome, such as stability and delivery method to the tumor cell.

Anti-Diabetes And Anti-Obesity Activities Of Bioactive Peptides

Recent research is revealing some exciting possible peptide therapies for diabetes and metabolic dysfunction. Metabolic syndrome involves a cluster of disorders such as insulin resistance, high blood pressure, and high cholesterol. Patients with metabolic syndrome have a sharply increased risk of heart attacks and developing diabetes. According to a 2020 study using computer modeling, five vegetable proteins derived from rice, chickpeas, and corn contain "cryptic" peptides which, when released by digestion or food processing, demonstrated "a high potential to be effective against metabolic syndrome." (Maldonado-Torres, 2020). These bioactive peptides could be included in future functional foods, foods which offer health benefits beyond their nutritional value.

Researchers recently investigated bioactive peptides with the ability to modify high blood pressure for their potential to address the problems of metabolic syndrome such as insulin resistance. Several drugs used to treat high blood pressure, called ACE inhibitors, have shown the capacity to improve several of the dysfunctional processes of metabolic syndrome. However, the scientists noted, the undesirable side effects of synthetic drugs have increased consumer interest in functional foods. Bioactive peptides with ACE-inhibitory properties have been studied extensively, and the effects of these antihypertensive peptides on other elements of metabolic syndrome are very encouraging. In tests with rats, bioactive peptides derived from dairy foods, eggs, and marine sources have improved insulin resistance, reduced inflammation in fat tissues, improved glucose tolerance, and reduced oxidative stress in endothelial cells. A freshly minted research review argues that peptides derived from eggs constitute "a new bioactive treasure for cardiometabolic diseases" such as Type 2 diabetes and metabolic syndrome (Moreno-Fernandez, 2020).

Another study showed that short peptides derived from collagen killed up to 80% of white adipose cells, the fat cells which stimulate the low-grade inflammation associated with obesity. Although in vivo human trials remain limited, patients with Type 2 diabetes who received a collagen peptide "showed marked improvements in fasting blood glucose,

HbAlc, and insulin sensitivity." (Sharkey, 2020). A clinical trial of human subjects with a peptide derived from skate skin showed reductions in body weight and fat mass. The authors of the review concluded that fish proteins provide peptides with great potential for clinical use in functional foods for the control of high blood sugar and excess body weight. Many of the same mechanisms associated with obesity, such as inflammation and oxidative stress, also contribute to premature aging.

Anti-Aging Effects Of Bioactive Peptides

Research teams around the world are investigating the clinical use of bioactive peptides to treat and reverse the physiological processes of aging. In April 2020, a study reported that a peptide derived from the sea cucumber is a potential anti-aging compound. It promoted longevity in fruit flies and reduced oxidative injury in mice. Scientists claimed that a sea cucumber peptide, AjPH, prolonged the survival of C. elegans nematodes exposed to oxidative stress in a study published in May 2020. AjPH directly scavenges free radicals and extends the nematode's lifespan and is a promising candidate for future anti-aging and antioxidant nutraceuticals.

Recent studies of collagen peptides continue to suggest that they possess significant anti-aging benefits in terms of skin elasticity, firmness, dryness, and wrinkling. A study published in January 2020, reported the results of a triple-blinded trial.

The trial was a study in which knowledge of the treatment assignment was concealed from the people who organized and analyzed the data as well as from subjects and investigators. The trial consisted of a food supplement containing special collagen peptides and other vitamins and nutrients which was taken by sixty women for twelve weeks. Images taken with a laser scanning microscope showed "significant improvement of the collagen structure of facial skin" in the women who took the supplement (Laing, 2020). Women who ingested the placebo showed no improvements. Similar results were achieved in a February 2020 study. Oral ingestion of collagen peptides increases skin moisture and elasticity, and topical application improves wrinkles, dryness, and skin firmness.

GHK, a naturally occurring peptide found in human serum, possesses significant anti-aging properties according to a study published in March 2020. Both GHK and GHK-Cu, copper peptide, have demonstrated antioxidant, anti-inflammatory, and skin remodeling and regeneration properties. GHK crosses the blood-brain barrier in rats and nonhuman primates. When administered to twenty eight-month-old mice (elderly, in mouse years), the mice performed significantly better in their ability to escape from a box maze than the control group which received a saline solution. The brain tissues of the GHK-treated mice showed less inflammation. Other indications suggested that the peptide also could be "triggering an epigenetic pathway in the amelioration of cognitive impairment in aging mice" (Dou, 2020). The study's authors concluded that the peptide could be included with other anti-aging drugs in a potent cocktail that would enhance health and extend life.

A drop in peptides produced in the mitochondria, the "powerhouses" of cells, has been linked with aging. One of these mitochondrial-derived peptides, humanin, was shown in a 2018 study to improve the cognitive abilities of aged mice and is linked with improved cognitive age in humans. In June 2020, the same research team reported that humanin did not just prevent age-related diseases, it also can increase the lifespan. Lower levels of humanin were associated with higher levels of disease, while higher levels of humanin were linked with longevity. Furthermore, they concluded that, "humanin, and perhaps other mitochondrial derived peptides, is not only correlated with health and lifespan but can significantly improve both parameters on its own" (Yen, 2020). A study published in September 2020, investigated how mitochondrial-derived peptides, humanin and MOTS-c, regulate key aging processes, including cognitive decline, chronic inflammation, and cellular senescence, or the inability of a cell to divide and replicate itself. Boosting levels of these peptides could have beneficial effects on several age-related dysfunctions.

Many bioactive peptides are currently in clinical trials for their beneficial effects on human health and longevity. So where can you learn more about these remarkable biomolecules and keep up with the latest developments about their life-enhancing, life-extending benefits?

Where To Learn More About Bioactive Peptides

You can visit www.Genostim.com to learn more about the Genostim® line of bioactive peptide products and www.TheGiftofLife.com to learn more about the Genostim® pet line of biopeptide products.

The future of bioactive peptide clinical applications and pharmaceuticals looks bright, with many promising new products in development. Genostim® Performance Labs will remain in the forefront of this exciting field and continue to provide you with the purest, naturally occurring, life-extending and life-enhancing bioactive peptides in all our products.

BIBLIOGRAPHY

Introduction

Bahar, Ali Adem and Dacheng Ren. "Antimicrobial Peptides." *Pharmaceuticals*, Vol. 6, No. 12, 18 November 2013: 1543–1575. https://www.ncbi.nlm.nih.gov/pmc/articles/PMC3873676/

Briquez, Priscilla S., Jeffrey A. Hubbell, and Mikaël M. Martino. "Extracellular Matrix-Inspired Growth Factor Delivery Systems for Skin Wound Healing." *Advances in Wound Care*, Vol. 4, No. 8, 2 Jul 2015. https://doi.org/10.1089/wound.2014.0603

Felman, Adam. "Who Discovered Insulin?" *Medical News Today*, 2018. https://www.medicalnewstoday.com/articles/323774

Findley, Fern et al. "Cationic Host Defense Peptides: Novel Antimicrobial Therapeutics Against Category A Pathogens and Emerging Infections." *Pathogens and Global Health*, Vol. 110, No. 4-5, June 2016: 137–147. https://doi: 10.1080/20477724.2016.1195036

Fitzpatrick, Richard E. and Elizabeth F. Rostan. "Reversal of Photodamage with Topical Growth Factors: A Pilot Study." *Journal of Cosmetic and Laser Therapy*, Vol. 5, No. 1, 2003: 25-34. https://doi.org/10.1080/14764170310000817

Haney, Evan F., Suzana K. Straus, and Robert E. W. Hancock. "Reassessing the Host Defense Peptide Landscape." *Frontiers in Chemistry*, 04 February 2019. https://doi.org/10.3389/fchem.2019.00043

Leslie, Mitch. "New Universe of Miniproteins is Upending Cell Biology and Genetics." *Science*, 17 October 2019. https://www.sciencemag.org/news/2019/10/new-universe-miniproteins-upending-cell-biology-and-genetics

Rosenfeld, Louis. "Insulin: Discovery and Controversy." *Clinical Chemistry*, Vol. 48, No. 12, 1 December 2002: 2270–2288. https://doi.org/10.1093/clinchem/48.12.2270

Rotwein, Peter. "Peptide Growth Factors," in *Endocrinology: Basic and Clinical Principles*, eds. P. Michael Conn and Shlomo Melmed. Totowa, NJ: Humana Press, 1997: 79 – 99. https://doi.org/10.1007/978-1-59259-641-6

Stokstad, Erik. "Sticky proteins could protect crops more safely than chemical pesticides." *Science*, Vol. 369, No. 6505, 14 August 2020. https://www.sciencemag.org/news/2019/04/sticky-proteins-could-protect-crops-more-safely-chemical-pesticides

Vecchio, Ignazio et al. "The Discovery of Insulin: An Important Milestone in the History of Medicine." *Frontiers in Endocrinology*, 23

October 2018. https://www.frontiersin.org/articles/10.3389/fendo.2018.00613/full

Wu, Douglas C. and Mitchel P. Goldman. "A Prospective, Randomized, Double-blind, Split-face Clinical Trial Comparing the Efficacy of Two Topical Human Growth Factors for the Rejuvenation of the Aging Face." *Journal of Clinical and Aesthetic Dermatology*, Vol. 10, No. 5, May 2017: 31–35. https://www.ncbi.nlm.nih.gov/pmc/articles/PMC5479475/

Chapter One

Ahrens, Sandra et al. "A Central Extended Amygdala Circuit That Modulates Anxiety." *Journal of Neuroscience* Vol. 38, No. 24, 13 June 2018: 5567-5583. https://doi.org/10.1523/JNEUROSCI.0705-18.2018.

Aloe, Luigi. "Nerve Growth Factor: From the Early Discoveries to the Potential Clinical Use." *Journal of Translational Medicine* Vol. 10, No. 239, 29 November 2012. https://translational-medicine.biomedcentral.com/articles/10.1186/1479-5876-10-239

Badenhorst, Travis et al. "Effects of GHK-Cu on MMP and TIMP Expression, Collagen and Elastin Production, and Facial Wrinkle Parameters." *Journal of Aging Science* Vol. 4, No. 3, 22 December 2016. https://doi.org/10.4172/2329-8847.1000166

Bahar, Ali Adem and Dacheng Ren. "Antimicrobial Peptides." *Pharmaceuticals*, Vol. 6, Issue 12, 18 November 2013: 1543–1575. https://www.ncbi.nlm.nih.gov/pmc/articles/PMC3873676/

Botelho, Mariana and Cláudia Cavadas. "Neuropeptide Y: An Anti-Aging Player?" *Trends in Neurosciences* Vol. 38, No. 11, 01 November 2015: 701-711. https://doi.org/10.1016/j.tins.2015.08.012

Charité - Universitätsmedizin Berlin. "An Interconnection Between the Nervous and Immune System: Neuroendocrine Reflex Triggers Infections." *Science Daily*, 19 September 2017. www.sciencedaily.com/releases/2017/09/170919102530.htm

Dou, Yan. "The Potential of GHK as an Anti-Aging Peptide." *Aging Pathobiology and Therapeutics* Vol. 2, No. 1, 2020:58-61. https://doi.org/10.31491/APT.2020.03.014

Dvorakova, Magdalena Chottova. "Distribution and Function of Neuropeptides W/B Signaling System." *Frontiers in Physiology*, 24 July 2018. https://doi.org/10.3389/fphys.2018.00981

Feng, Yuan et al. "Current Research on Opioid Receptor Function." *Current Drug Targets* Vol. 13, No. 2, Feb 2012: 230-246. https://www.ncbi.nlm.nih.gov/pmc/articles/PMC3371376/

Henry, Mathilde S. et al. "Enkephalins: Endogenous Analgesics with an Emerging Role in Stress Resilience." *Neural Plasticity*, 11 July 2017. https://doi.org/10.1155/2017/1546125

Holloway, Marguerite. "Finding the Good in the Bad: A Profile of Rita Levi-Montalcini." *Scientific American*, 30 December 2012. https://www.scientificamerican.com/article/finding-the-good-rita-levi-montalcini/

Hou, Gang and Xiaoming Zhou. "Antioxidant and Anti-Inflammation Effect of GHK-Cu in Bleomycin-Induced Pulmonary Fibrosis." *European Respiratory Journal* Vo. 52, No. 62, 2018: 2957. https://doi.org/10.1183/13993003.congress-2018.PA2957

Li, Qin, Aundrea F. Bartley and Lynn E. Dobrunz. "Endogenously Released Neuropeptide Y Suppresses Hippocampal Short-Term Facilitation and Is Impaired by Stress-Induced Anxiety." *Journal of Neuroscience* Vol. 37, No. 1, 4 January 2017: 23-37. https://doi.org/10.1523/JNEUROSCI.2599-16.2016

McDonald, Marguerite B. "Topical Recombinant Human Nerve Growth Factor an Innovation in Ocular Surface Disease Treatment." *Ocular Surgery News*, 12 October 2018. https://www.healio.com/news/ophthalmology/20181010/topical-recombinant-human-nerve-growth-factor-an-innovation-in-ocular-surface-disease-treatment

Noble, Emily E. et al. "Control of Feeding Behavior by Cerebral Ventricular Volume Transmission of Melanin-Concentrating Hormone." *Cell Metabolism* Vol. 28, No. 1, 3

July 2018: 55-68.37. https://doi.org/10.1016/j.cmet.2018.05.001

Oh, Tae Seok et al. "Hypothalamic AMPK-induced Autophagy Increases Food Intake by Regulating NPY and POMC Expression." *Autophagy*, Vol. 12, No. 11: 2009–2025 (2016). https://doi.org/10.1080/15548627.2016.1215382

Okamura, Naoe et al. "Neuropeptide S Enhances Memory During the Consolidation Phase and Interacts with Noradrenergic Systems in the Brain." *Neuropsychopharmacology* Vol. 36, No. 4, March 2011: 744–752. https://www.ncbi.nlm.nih.gov/pmc/articles/PMC3037424/

Palamiuc, Lavinia et al. "A Tachykinin-Like Neuroendocrine Signalling Axis Couples Central Serotonin Action and Nutrient Sensing With Peripheral Lipid Metabolism." *Nature Communications* 8, 14237 (2017). https://doi.org/10.1038/ncomms14237

Pickart, Loren and Anna Margolina. "Regenerative and Protective Actions of the GHK-Cu Peptide in the Light of the New Gene Data." *International Journal of Molecular Sciences* Vol. 19, No. 7, 7 July 2018. *https://doi.org/10.3390/ijms19071987*

——, Jessica Michelle Vasquez-Soltero, and Anna Margolina. "The Human Tripeptide GHK-Cu in Prevention of Oxidative Stress and Degenerative Conditions of Aging: Implications for Cognitive Health." *Oxidative*

Medicine and Cellular Longevity 10 May 2012. https://doi.org/10.1155/2012/324832

Sánchez, Adrián, and Alfredo Vázquez. "Bioactive Peptides: A Review." *Food Quality and Safety*, Volume 1, No. 1, 1 March 2017: 29–46. https://doi.org/10.1093/fqsafe/fyx006

Singh, Gurminder and Anthony P Davenport. "Neuropeptide B and W: Neurotransmitters in an Emerging G-Protein-Coupled Receptor System." *British Journal of Pharmacology* Vol. 148, No. 8, August 2006:1033–1041. https://doi.org/10.1038/sj.bjp.0706825

Sporn, Michael B. and Anita B. Roberts. "Peptide Growth Factors and Inflammation, Tissue Repair, and Cancer." *Journal of Clinical Investigation* Vol. 78, No. 2, August 1986: 329–332. https://doi.org/10.1172/JCI112580

Sprouse-Blum, Adam S. et al. "Understanding Endorphins and Their Importance in Pain Management." *Hawai'i Medical Journal* Vol 69, No. 3, March 2010: 70–71. https://www.ncbi.nlm.nih.gov/pmc/articles/PMC3104618/#

Wang, Xinying et al. "GHK-Cu-Liposomes Accelerate Scald Wound Healing in Mice by Promoting Cell Proliferation and Angiogenesis." *Wound Repair and Regeneration* Vol. 25, No. 2, March/April 2017: 270-278. https://doi.org/10.1111/wrr.12520

Winter, Patricia de, Patricia Leoni, and David Abraham. "Connective Tissue Growth Factor: Structure-Function Relationships of a Mosaic,

Multifunctional Protein." *Growth Factors* Vol. 26, No. 2, April 2008: 80-91. https://doi.org/10.1080/08977190802025602

Xu, Xin et al. "Transforming Growth Factor-β in Stem Cells and Tissue Homeostasis." *Bone Research* Volume 6, No. 2, 31 January 2018. https://www.nature.com/articles/s41413-017-0005-4

Yi, Min et al. "A Promising Therapeutic Target for Metabolic Diseases: Neuropeptide Y Receptors in Humans." *Cellular Physiology and Biochemistry* Vol. 45, 2018: 88–107. https://doi.org/10.1159/000486225

Yun, Ye-Rang et al. "Fibroblast Growth Factors: Biology, Function, and Application for Tissue Regeneration." *Journal of Tissue Engineering* Vol. 2010, No. 218142, 7 November 2010. https://doi.org/10.4061/2010/218142

Chapter Two

Agyei, Dominic, Ravichandra Potumarthi, and Michael K. Danquah. "Food-Derived Multifunctional Bioactive Proteins and Peptides: Sources and Production," in *Biotechnology of Bioactive Compounds: Sources and Applications*. Eds. Vijai Kumar Gupta et al. John Wiley & Sons, 2015: 483-505.

Albenzio, Marzia. "Bioactive Peptides in Animal Food Products." *Foods* Vol. 6, No. 35, 2017. https://doi.org/10.3390/foods6050035

Amigo, Lourdes, Daniel Martínez-Maqueda, and Blanca Hernández-Ledesma. "In Silico and In Vitro Analysis of Multifunctionality of Animal Food-Derived Peptides." *Foods* Vol. 9, No. 8, 24 July 2020. https://doi.org/10.3390/foods9080991

Aneiros, Abel and Anoland Garateix. "Bioactive Peptides From Marine Sources: Pharmacological Properties and Isolation Procedures." *Journal of Chromatography B*, Vol. 803, 2004: 41–53. https://doi.org/doi:10.1016/j.jchromb.2003.11.005

Arsenault, Chris. "Only 60 Years of Farming Left If Soil Degradation Continues." *Scientific American*, 5 December 2014. https://www.scientificamerican.com/article/only-60-years-of-farming-left-if-soil-degradation-continues/

Bhat, Z.F. and Sunil Kumar. "Bioactive Peptides From Egg: A Review." *Nutrition and Food Science* Vol. 45, No. 2, 2015: 190-2012. https://doi.org/10.1108/NFS-10-2014-0088

Chen, Ying-Lan. "The Role of Peptides Cleaved From Protein Precursors in Eliciting Plant Stress Reactions." *New Phytologist* Vol. 225, No. 6, March 2020: 2267-2282. https://doi.org/10.1111/nph.16241

Cosier, Susan. "The World Needs Topsoil to Grow 95% of Its Food – But It's Rapidly Disappearing." *The Guardian*, 30 May 2019. https://www.

theguardian.com/us-news/2019/may/30/top-soil-farming-agriculture-food-toxic-america

Dávalos, Alberto, Marta Miguel, and R López-Fandiño. "Antioxidant Activity of Peptides Derived from Egg White Proteins by Enzymatic Hydrolysis." *Journal of Food Protection* Vol. 67, No. 9, October 2004: 1939-44. https://doi.org/10.4315/0362-028X-67.9.1939

DeMartini, Alayna. "Higher Carbon Dioxide Levels Prompt More Plant Growth, But Fewer Nutrients." 3 April 2018. Ohio State University College of Food, Agricultural, and Environmental Sciences. https://cfaes.osu.edu/news/articles/higher-carbon-dioxide-levels-prompt-more-plant-growth-fewer-nutrients

Eckert, Ewelina et al. "Biologically Active Peptides Derived From Egg Proteins." *World's Poultry Science Journal* Vol. 69, June 2013. https://doi.org/10.101 7/S0043 93391300 0366

Escudero, Elizabeth. "Identification of Novel Antioxidant Peptides Generated in Spanish Dry-Cured Ham." *Food Chemistry* Vol. 138, No. 2-3, 1 June 2013: 1282-8. https://doi.org/10.1016/j.foodchem.2012.10.133.

Esfandi, Ramak, Mallory E. Walters, and Apollinaire Tsopmo. "Antioxidant Properties and Potential Mechanisms of Hydrolyzed Proteins and Peptides From Cereals." *Heliyon* Vol. 5, 2019. https://doi.org/10.1016/j.heliyon.2019.e01538

Fukudome, Shin-ichi and Masaaki Yoshikawa. "Opioid Peptides Derived From Wheat Gluten: Their Isolation and Characterization." *FEBS Letters* Vol. 296, No. 1, January 1992: 107-111. https://doi.org/10.1016/0014-5793(92)80414-c

Gao, Ruichang et al. "Sturgeon Protein-Derived Peptides Exert Anti-Inflammatory Effects in LPS-Stimulated RAW264.7 Macrophages Via The MAPK Pathway." *Journal of Functional Foods* Vo. 72, September 2020. https://doi.org/10.1016/j.jff.2020.104044

Ghorbani, Sarieh. "Signaling Peptides in Plants." *Cell and Developmental Biology* Vol. 3, No. 2, 2014. https://doi.org/10.4172/2168-9296.1000141

González-Montoya, Marcela, Eden Cano-Sampedro and Rosalva Mora-Escobedo. "Bioactive Peptides from Legumes as Anticancer Therapeutic Agents." *International Journal of Cancer and Clinical Research* Vol. 4, No. 2, 19 July 2017. https://doi.org/10.23937/2378-3419/1410081

Kennedy, Merrit. "As Carbon Dioxide Levels Rise, Major Crops Are Losing Nutrients." *NPR*, 19 June 2018. https://www.npr.org/sections/the-salt/2018/06/19/616098095/as-carbon-dioxide-levels-rise-major-crops-are-losing-nutrients

Lafarga, Tomas and Maria Hayes. "Bioactive Peptides From Meat Muscle and By-Products: Generation, Functionality and Application as Functional Ingredients." *Meat Science* Vol.

98, No. 2, October 2014: 227-39. https://doi.org/10.1016/j.meatsci.2014.05.036

Liu, Dongmei et al. "Generation of Bioactive Peptides From Duck Meat During Post-Mortem Aging." *Food Chemistry* Vol. 237, 15 December 2017: 408-415. https://doi.org/10.1016/j.foodchem.2017.05.094

Madureira, A.R. et al. "Physiological Properties of Bioactive Peptides Obtained From Whey Proteins." *Journal of Dairy Science* Vol. 93, 2010: 437-455. https://doi.org/10.3168/jds.2009-2566

Maestri, Elena et al. "Meta-Analysis for Correlating Structure of Bioactive Peptides in Foods of Animal Origin with Regard to Effect and Stability." *Comprehensive Reviews in Food Science and Food Safety* Vol. 18, No. 1, January 2019: 3-30. https://doi.org/10.1111/1541-4337.12402

Ryan, Joseph Thomas et al. "Bioactive Peptides from Muscle Sources: Meat and Fish." *Nutrients* Vol. 3, No. 9, September 2011: 765–791. https://doi.org/10.3390/nu3090765

Sánchez, Adrián, and Alfredo Vázquez. "Bioactive Peptides: A Review." *Food Quality and Safety*, Volume 1, No. 1, 1 March 2017: 29–46. https://doi.org/10.1093/fqsafe/fyx006

Scheer, Roddy and Doug Moss. "Dirt Poor: Have Fruits and Vegetables Become Less Nutritious?" *Scientific American*, 27 April

2011. https://www.scientificamerican.com/article/soil-depletion-and-nutrition-loss/

Scheier, Lee M. "What Is the Hunger-Obesity Paradox?" *Journal of the Academy of Nutrition and Dietetics*, Vol. 105, No. 6, June 2005: 883-886. https://doi.org/10.1016/j.jada.2005.04.013

Suglia, Elena. "Vanishing Nutrients." *Scientific American*, 10 December 2018. https://blogs.scientificamerican.com/observations/vanishing-nutrients/

Tsuruoka, Nobuo. "A DKP Cyclo(L-Phe-L-Phe) Found in Chicken Essence Is a Dual Inhibitor of the Serotonin Transporter and Acetylcholinesterase." PLoS One Vol. 7, No. 11, 28 November 2012. https://doi.org/10.1371/journal.pone.0050824

Watts, Jonathan. "Third of Earth's Soil is Acutely Degraded Due to Agriculture." *The Guardian*, 12 September 2017. https://www.theguardian.com/environment/2017/sep/12/third-of-earths-soil-acutely-degraded-due-to-agriculture-study

Wu, Dan et al. "Structure-Activity Relationship and Pathway of Antioxidant Shrimp Peptides in a PC12 Cell Model." *Journal of Functional Foods* Vol. 70, July 2020. https://doi.org/10.1016/j.jff.2020.103978

Xing, Lujuan. "Meat Protein Based Bioactive Peptides and Their Potential Functional Activity: A Review." *International Journal of Food Science and Technology* Vol. 54, No. 6, June 2019: 1956-1966. https://doi.org/10.1111/ijfs.14132

Zhu, Chunwu et al. "Carbon Dioxide (CO 2) Levels This Century Will Alter the Protein, Micronutrients, and Vitamin Content of Rice Grains With Potential Health Consequences for the Poorest Rice-Dependent Countries." *Science Advances* Vol. 4, No. 5, May 2018. https://doi.org/10.1126/sciadv.aaq1012

Ziska, Lewis H. et al. "Rising Atmospheric CO2 is Reducing the Protein Concentration of a Floral Pollen Source Essential for North American Bees." *Proceedings of the Royal Society B*, Vol. 283, No. 1828, 13 April 2016. https://doi.org/10.1098/rspb.2016.0414

Chapter Three

Anisimov, Vladimir N., Alexander V. Arutjunyan, and Vladimir Kh. Khavinson. "Effects of Pineal Peptide Preparation Epithalamin on Free-Radical Processes in Humans and Animals." *Neuroendocrinology Letters* Vol. 22, No. 1, 2001:9 –18. https://pubmed.ncbi.nlm.nih.gov/11335874/

Bayliss, W.M. and E.H. Starling, "The Mechanism of Pancreatic Secretion." *Journal of Physiology* Vol. 18, 1902: 325-353. https://www.ncbi.nlm.nih.gov/pmc/articles/PMC1665254/bin/jphysiol_2004.073056_1.pdf

Hench, Philip S. et al. "Effect of Cortisone and Pituitary Adrenocorticotropic Hormone (ACTH) On Rheumatic Diseases." *Journal of American Medical Association* No. 144, No. 16, 16 December 1950:1327-1335. https://doi.org/10.1001/jama.1950.02920160001001

Henderson, John. "Ernest Starling and 'Hormones': An Historical Commentary." *Journal of Endocrinology* Vol. 184, No. 1, 205: 5-10. https://doi.org/10.1677/joe.1.06000

Hirst, Barry M. "Secretin and the Exposition of Hormonal Control." *Journal of Physiology* Vol. 560(Pt 2), 15 October 2004: 339. https://doi.org/10.1113/jphysiol.2004.073056

Karpova, Lisa. "Live to 100 Says Russian Physician." *Pravda.ru*, 10 October 2011. https://www.pravdareport.com/health/119286-Live_to_100_says_Russian_physician/

Khavinson, Vladimir. "Peptide Regulation of Ageing." N.d. https://khavinson.info/research/peptide-regulation-of-ageing

—— et al. "AEDG Peptide (Epitalon) Stimulates Gene Expression and Protein Synthesis during Neurogenesis: Possible Epigenetic Mechanism." *Molecules* Vol. 25, No. 3, 30 January 2020:609. https://doi.org/10.3390/molecules25030609.

—— et al. "GDF11 Protein as a Geroprotector." *Biology Bulletin Reviews* Vol. 6, 16 May 2016: 141–148. https://doi.org/10.1134/S207908641602002X

——, B. I. Kuznik and G. A. Ryzhak. “Peptide bioregulators: A New Class of Geroprotectors, Report 2. The Results of Clinical Trials.” *Advances in Gerontology* Vol. 4, No. 4, 2014: 346-361.

—— and Vladimir N. Anisimov. “Peptide Regulation of Aging: 35-Year Research Experience.” *Bulletin of Experimental Biology and Medicine* Vol. 148, No. 1, July 2009: 94-99. https://doi.org/10.1007/s10517-009-0650-8

—— and Vyacheslav Morozov. “Peptides of Pineal Gland and Thymus Prolong Human Life.” *Neuroendocrinology Letters* Vol. 24, No. 3-4, 2003: 233-240.

Korkushko, Oleg Vasilevich et al. “Peptide Geroprotector from the Pituitary Gland Inhibits Rapid Aging of Elderly People: Results of 15-Year Follow-Up.” *Bulletin of Experimental Biology and Medicine* Vol. 151, 2011: 366–369. https://doi.org/10.1007/s10517-011-1332-x

Lau, Jolene L. and Michael K. Dunn. “Therapeutic Peptides: Historical Perspectives, Current Development Trends, and Future Directions.” *Bioorganic and Medicinal Chemistry*, Vol. 26, 2018: 2700-2707. https://doi.org/10.1016/j.bmc.2017.06.052

Linkova, Natalia S., B.I. Kuznik and Vladimir Khavinson. “The Peptide Ala-Glu-Asp-Gly and Interferon Gamma: Their Role in Immune Response During Aging.” *Advances in*

Gerontology Vol. 3, April 2013: 124-128. https://doi.org/10.1134/S2079057013020100

Micans, Philip. "The Remarkable Role of Peptide Bioregulators for Human Health." *AgingMatters Magazine*, 29 November 2016. https://aging-matters.com/the-remarkable-role-of-peptide-bioregulators-for-human-health/

Rattan, Suresh I. S. ""I Think That the Small Peptides Are the Best for Healthy Ageing': An Interview With Vladimir Khavinson." *Biogerontology* Vol. 14, January 2013:1–8. https://doi.org/10.1007/s10522-013-9414-y

Chapter Four

Asserin, Jérome. "The Effect of Oral Collagen Peptide Supplementation on Skin Moisture and the Dermal Collagen Network: Evidence From an Ex Vivo Model and Randomized, Placebo-Controlled Clinical Trials." *Journal of Cosmetic Dermatology* Vol. 14, No. 4, December 2015: 291-301. https://doi.org/10.1111/jocd.12174

Baar, Marjolein P. "Targeted Apoptosis of Senescent Cells Restores Tissue Homeostasis in Response to Chemotoxicity and Aging." *Cell* Vol. 169, No. 1, 23 March 2017: 132-147.e16. https://doi.org/10.1016/j.cell.2017.02.031

Cell Press. "Peptide Targeting Senescent Cells Restores Stamina, Fur, And Kidney

Function In Old Mice." *Science Daily*, 23 March 2017. <www.sciencedaily.com/releases/2017/03/170323141414.htm>

Cobb, Laura J. et al. "Naturally Occurring Mitochondrial-Derived Peptides Are Age-Dependent Regulators of Apoptosis, Insulin Sensitivity, and Inflammatory Markers." *Aging* Vol. 8, No. 4, April 2016: 796-809. https://doi.org/10.18632/aging.100943

Farr, Joshua N. et al. "Targeting Cellular Senescence Prevents Age-Related Bone Loss in Mice." *Nature Medicine* Vol. 23, 21 August 2017: 1072-1079. https://doi.org/10.1038/nm.4385

Felician, Fatuma Felix et al. "The Wound Healing Potential of Collagen Peptides Derived from the Jellyfish *Rhopilema Esculentum*." *Chinese Journal of Traumatology* Vol. 22, No. 1, February 2019: 12-20. https://doi.org/10.1016/j.cjtee.2018.10.004

De Keiser, Peter L.J. "The Fountain of Youth by Targeting Senescent Cells?" *Trends in Molecular Medicine* Vol. 23, No. 1, 1 January 2017: 6-17. https://doi.org/10.1016/j.molmed.2016.11.006

Hu, Zhang et al. "Marine Collagen Peptides from the Skin of Nile Tilapia (Oreochromis niloticus): Characterization and Wound Healing Evaluation." *Marine Drugs* Vol. 15, No. 4, April 2017: 102. https://doi.org/10.3390/md15040102

Inoue, Naoki, Fumihito Sugihara and Xuemin Wan. "Ingestion of Bioactive Collagen Hydrolysates Enhance Facial Skin Moisture and Elasticity and Reduce Facial Ageing Signs in a Randomised Double-Blind Placebo-Controlled Clinical Study." *Journal of the Science of Food and Agriculture* Vol. 96, No. 12, September 2016: 4077-81. https://doi.org/10.1002/jsfa.7606

Jendricke, Patrick et al. "Specific Collagen Peptides in Combination with Resistance Training Improve Body Composition and Regional Muscle Strength in Premenopausal Women: A Randomized Controlled Trial." *Nutrients* Vol. 11, No. 4, April 2019: 892. https://doi.org/10.3390/nu11040892

Kim, Do-Un et al. "Oral Intake of Low-Molecular-Weight Collagen Peptide Improves Hydration, Elasticity, and Wrinkling in Human Skin: A Randomized, Double-Blind, Placebo-Controlled Study." *Nutrients* Vol. 10, No. 7, July 2018: 826. https://doi.org/10.3390/nu10070826

Kimse, Marius et al. "Prolonged Collagen Peptide Supplementation and Resistance Exercise Training Affects Body Composition in Recreationally Active Men." *Nutrients* Vol. 11, No. 5, May 2019: 1154. https://doi.org/10.3390/nu11051154

König, Daniel et al. "Specific Collagen Peptides Improve Bone Mineral Density and Bone

Markers in Postmenopausal Women—A Randomized Controlled Study." *Nutrients* Vol 10, No. 1, January 2018: 97. https://doi.org/10.3390/nu10010097

Lau, Jolene L. and Michael K. Dunn. "Therapeutic Peptides: Historical Perspectives, Current Development Trends, and Future Directions." *Bioorganic and Medicinal Chemistry*, Vol. 26, 2018: 2700-2707. https://doi.org/10.1016/j.bmc.2017.06.052

Mei, Fengfeng et al. "Collagen Peptides Isolated from Salmo salar and Tilapia nilotica Skin Accelerate Wound Healing by Altering Cutaneous Microbiome Colonization via Upregulated NOD2 and BD14." *Journal of Agricultural and Food Chemistry* Vol. 68, No. 6, 22 January 2020: 1621-1633. https://doi.org/10.1021/acs.jafc.9b08002

Mistry, Krishan et al. "Promoting Cutaneous Wound Healing With Nutraceutical Porcine Type I Collagen Peptides." *Journal of Investigative Dermatology* Vol. 140, No. 7, July 2020: S104. https://doi.org/10.1016/j.jid.2020.03.806

Mu, Lixian et al. "A Potential Wound-Healing-Promoting Peptide from Salamander Skin." *The FASEB Journal* Vol. 28, No. 9, September 2014: 3919–3929. https://doi.org/10.1096/fj.13-248476

Peng, Xue et al. "Marine Fish Peptides (Collagen Peptides) Compound Intake Promotes Wound

Healing in Rats after Cesarean Section." *Food & Nutrition Research* Vol. 64, 31 August 2020. https://doi.org/10.29219/fnr.v64.4247

Proksch, Ehrhardt et al. "Oral Intake of Specific Bioactive Collagen Peptides Reduces Skin Wrinkles and Increases Dermal Matrix Synthesis." *Skin Pharmacology and Physiology* Vol. 27, No. 3, 2014: 113-119. https://doi.org/10.1159/000355523

———. "Oral Supplementation of Specific Collagen Peptides Has Beneficial Effects on Human Skin Physiology: A Double-Blind, Placebo-Controlled Study." *Skin Pharmacology and Physiology* Vol. 27, No. 1, 2014: 47-55. https://doi.org/10.1159/000351376

Subbotina, Ekaterina et al. "Musclin is an Activity-Stimulated Myokine That Enhances Physical Endurance." *Proceedings of the National Academy of Sciences* Vol. 112, No. 52, 29 December 2015:16042-7 https://doi.org/10.1073/pnas.1514250112.

Uehara, Takashi et al. "Delivery of RANKL-Binding Peptide OP3-4 Promotes BMP-2-Induced Maxillary Bone Regeneration." *Journal of Dental Research* Vol. 95, No. 6, June 2016: 665-72. https://doi.org/10.1177/0022034516633170

Wang, Lin et al. "Effect of Oral Administration of Collagen Hydrolysates from Nile Tilapia on the Chronologically Aged Skin." *Journal of*

Functional Foods Vol. 44, May 2018: 112-117. https://doi.org/10.1016/j.jff.2018.03.005

Yen, Kelvin et al. "The Mitochondrial Derived Peptide Humanin Is a Regulator of Lifespan and Healthspan." *Aging* Vol. 12, No. 12, 23 June 2020:11185-11199. https://doi.org/10.18632/aging.103534.

——. "Humanin Prevents Age-Related Cognitive Decline in Mice and is Associated with Improved Cognitive Age in Humans." *Scientific Reports* Vol. 8, Article No.: 14212. 21 September 2018. https://doi.org/10.1038/s41598-018-32616-7

Zdzieblik, Denise et al. "Collagen Peptide Supplementation in Combination with Resistance Training Improves Body Composition and Increases Muscle Strength in Elderly Sarcopenic Men: A Randomised Controlled Trial." *British Journal of Nutrition* Vol. 114, No. 8, 28 October 2015: 1237–1245. https://doi.org/10.1017/S0007114515002810

Chapter Five

Agarwal, Garima and Reema Gabrani. "Antiviral Peptides: Identification and Validation." *International Journal of Peptide Research and Therapeutics*, 18 May 2020 May: 1-20. https://doi.org/10.1007/s10989-020-10072-0.

Augustin, René et al. "Activity of the Novel Peptide Arminin against Multiresistant Human

Pathogens Shows the Considerable Potential of Phylogenetically Ancient Organisms as Drug Sources." *Antimicrobial Agents and Chemotherapy* Vol. 53, No. 12, December 2009: 5245–5250. https://doi.org/10.1128/AAC.00826-09

Bartels, Emiel Jacob Henri, Douwe Dekker and Mohamed Amiche. "Dermaseptins, Multifunctional Antimicrobial Peptides: A Review of Their Pharmacology, Effectivity, Mechanism of Action, and Possible Future Directions." *Frontiers in Pharmacology*, 26 November 2019. https://doi.org/10.3389/fphar.2019.01421

Brady, Daniel et al. "Insect Cecropins, Antimicrobial Peptides with Potential Therapeutic Applications." *International Journal of Molecular Sciences* Vol. 20, No. 23, 22 November 2019:5862. https://doi.org/10.3390/ijms20235862.

Braff, M.H. and Richard L. Gallo. "Antimicrobial Peptides: An Essential Component of the Skin Defensive Barrier." *Current Topics in Microbiology and Immunology* Vol. 306, 2006: 91-110. https://doi.org/10.1007/3-540-29916-5_4

Campione, Elena et al. "Lactoferrin as Protective Natural Barrier of Respiratory and Intestinal Mucosa against Coronavirus Infection and Inflammation." *International Journal of Molecular Sciences* Vol. 21, No. 14, 11

July 2020: 4903. https://doi.org/10.3390/ijms21144903

Coates, Margaret, Sarah Blanchard, and Amanda S. MacLeod. "Innate Antimicrobial Immunity in the Skin: A Protective Barrier against Bacteria, Viruses, and Fungi." *PLOS Pathogens* Vol. 14, No. 12, 6 December 2018: e1007353. 10.1371/journal.ppat.1007353

Conlon, J. Michael et al. "Host-Defense Peptides in Skin Secretions of the Tetraploid Frog Silurana Epitropicalis with Potent Activity Against Methicillin-Resistant Staphylococcus Aureus (MRSA)." *Peptides* Vol. 37, No. 1, September 2012: 113-119. https://doi.org/10.1016/j.peptides.2012.07.005

De Lucca, Anthony J. and Thomas J. Walsh. "Antifungal Peptides: Novel Therapeutic Compounds against Emerging Pathogens." *Antimicrobial Agents and Chemotherapy* Vol. 43, No. 1, January 1999: 1-11. https://doi.org/10.1128/AAC.43.1.1

De Ullivarri, Miguel Fernández et al. "Antifungal Peptides as Therapeutic Agents." *Frontiers in Cellular and Infection Microbiology* Vol. 10, 17 March 2020: 105. https://doi.org/10.3389/fcimb.2020.00105

De la Fuente-Núñez, César et al. "Broad-Spectrum Anti-biofilm Peptide That Targets a Cellular Stress Response." *PLOS Pathogens* Vo. 10, No. 5, May 2014. https://doi.org/10.1371/journal.ppat.1004152

Dhople, Vishnu, Amy Krukemeyer, and Ayyalusamy Ramamoorthy. "The Human Beta-Defensin-3, an Antibacterial Peptide with Multiple Biological Functions." *Biochimica et Biophysica Acta (BBA) – Biomembranes* Vol. 1758, No. 9, September 2006: 1499-1512. https://doi.org/10.1016/j.bbamem.2006.07.007

Dürr, Ulrich H.N., U.S. Sudheendra and AyyalusamyRamamoorthy. "LL-37, the Only Human Member of the Cathelicidin Family of Antimicrobial Peptides." *Biochimica et Biophysica Acta (BBA) – Biomembranes* Vol. 1758, No. 9, September 2006: 1408-1425. https://doi.org/10.1016/j.bbamem.2006.03.030

Elnagdy, Sherif and Maha AlKhazindar. "The Potential of Antimicrobial Peptides as an Antiviral Therapy against COVID-19." *ACS Pharmacology and Translational Science* Vol. 3, No. 4, 16 June 2020: 780–782. https://doi.org/10.1021/acsptsci.0c00059

Fakih, Taufik Muhammad. "Dermaseptin-Based Antiviral Peptides to Prevent COVID-19 through In Silico Molecular Docking Studies against SARS-CoV-2 Spike Protein." *Pharmaceutical Sciences and Research* Vol. 7, No. 4, 2020. https://doi.org/10.7454/psr.v7i4.1079

Findley, Fern et al. "Cationic Host Defense Peptides: Novel Antimicrobial Therapeutics Against Category A Pathogens and Emerging

Infections." *Pathogens and Global Health* Vol. 110 (4-5) June 2016: 137–147. https://doi.org/10.1080/20477724.2016.1195036

Gomes da Mata, Élida Cleyse et al. "Antiviral Activity of Animal Venom Peptides and Related Compounds." *Journals of Venomous Animals and Toxins including Tropical Diseases* Vol. 23, 2013: 3. https://doi.org/10.1186/s40409-016-0089-0

Hancock, Robert E.W., Evan F. Haney and Erin E. Gill. "The Immunology of Host Defence Peptides: Beyond Antimicrobial Activity." *Nature Reviews Immunology* Vol. 16, No. 5, May 2016 May:321-34 https://doi.org/10.1038/nri.2016.29.

Haney, Evan F., Suzana K. Straus and Robert E. W. Hancock. "Reassessing the Host Defense Peptide Landscape." *Frontiers in Chemistry* 04 February 2019. https://doi.org/10.3389/fchem.2019.00043

Hebbar, Nikhil. "Naturally Generated Decoy of the Prostate Apoptosis Response-4 Protein Overcomes Therapy Resistance in Tumors." *Cancer Research* Vol. 77, No. 15, 1 August 2017: 4039-4050. https://doi.org/10.1158/0008-5472.CAN-16-1970

Hoffmann, Andrew R. "Broad-Spectrum Antiviral Entry Inhibition by Interfacially-Active Peptides." *Journal of Virology*, 9 September 2020. https://doi.org/10.1128/JVI.01682-20

Holthausen, David J. et al. "An Amphibian Host Defense Peptide Is Virucidal for Human H1 Hemagglutinin-Bearing Influenza Viruses." *Immunity* Vol. 46, 18 April 2017: 587–595. https://doi.org/10.1016/j.immuni.2017.03.018

Luteijn, Rutger D. et al. "A Broad-Spectrum Antiviral Peptide Blocks Infection of Viruses by Binding to Phosphatidylserine in the Viral Envelope." *Cells* Vol. 9, No. 9, 29 August 2020: 1989. https://doi.org/10.3390/cells9091989

Mahlapuu, Margit et al. "Antimicrobial Peptides: An Emerging Category of Therapeutic Agents." *Frontiers in Cellular and Infection Microbiology* 27 December 2016. https://doi.org/10.3389/fcimb.2016.00194.

Maiti, Biplab K. "Potential Role of Peptide-Based Antiviral Therapy Against SARS-CoV-2 Infection." *ACS Pharmacology and Translational Science* Vol. 3, No. 4, 24 July 2020: 783–785. https://doi.org/10.1021/acsptsci.0c00081

Meade, Kieran G. and Cliona O'Farrelly. "β-Defensins: Farming the Microbiome for Homeostasis and Health." Frontiers in Immunology, Vol. 9, 25 January 2018: 3072. https://doi.org/10.3389/fimmu.2018.03072

Mookherjee, Neeloffer et al. "Antimicrobial Host Defence Peptides: Functions and Clinical Potential." *Nature Reviews Drug Discovery* Vol. 19, May 2020: 311–332. https://doi.org/10.1038/s41573-019-0058-8

Pan, W-R. et al. "Bovine Lactoferricin B Induces Apoptosis of Human Gastric Cancer Cell Line AGS by Inhibition of Autophagy at a Late Stage." *Journal of Dairy Science* Vol. 96, no. 12, December 2013: 7511-7520. https://doi.org/10.3168/jds.2013-7285

Rivas-Santiago, Bruno et al. "Ability of Innate Defence Regulator Peptides IDR-1002, IDR-HH2 and IDR-1018 to Protect against Mycobacterium tuberculosis Infections in Animal Models." *PLoS One* Vol. 8, No. 3, 21 Mar 2013: e59119. https://doi.org/10.1371/journal.pone.0059119

Samgina, Tatiana Yu et al. "Composition and Antimicrobial Activity of the Skin Peptidome of Russian Brown Frog Rana temporaria." *Journal of Proteome Research* Vol. 11, No. 12, 7 December 2012: 5573-6294. https://doi.org/10.1021/pr300890m

Scott, Monisha G. et al. "The Human Antimicrobial Peptide LL-37 Is a Multifunctional Modulator of Innate Immune Responses." *The Journal of Immunology* Vol. 169, No. 7, November 2002: 3883-91. . https://doi.org/10.4049/jimmunol.169.7.3883

Scudiero, Olga et al. "Human Defensins: A Novel Approach in the Fight against Skin Colonizing Staphylococcus aureus." *Antibiotics* Vol. 9, No. 4, 21 April 2020: 198. https://doi.org/10.3390/antibiotics9040198

Smith, Jason G. and Glen R. Nemerow. "Mechanism of Adenovirus Neutralization by Human α-Defensins." *Cell Host and Microbe* Vol. 3, No. 1, 17 January 2008: 11-19. https://doi.org/10.1016/j.chom.2007.12.001

Song, Chen et al. "Crystal Structure and Functional Mechanism of a Human Antimicrobial Membrane Channel." *Proceedings of the National Academy of Sciences* Vol. 110, No. 12, 19 March 2013:4586-91. https://doi.org/10.1073/pnas.1214739110

Soto-Pantoja, David R. et al. "Angiotensin-(1-7) Inhibits Tumor Angiogenesis in Human Lung Cancer Xenografts with a Reduction in Vascular Endothelial Growth Factor." *Molecular Cancer Therapeutics* Vol. 8, No. 6, June 2009: 1676–1683. https://doi.org/10.1158/1535-7163.MCT-09-0161

Steinstraesser, Lars et al. "Host Defense Peptides in Wound Healing." *Molecular Medicine* Vol. 14, 26 March 2008: 528–537. https://doi.org/10.2119/2008-00002.Steinstraesser

Uccelletti, Daniela et al. "Anti-Pseudomonas activity of Frog Skin Antimicrobial Peptides in a *Caenorhabditis Elegans* Infection Model: A Plausible Mode Of Action in Vitro and in Vivo." *Antimicrobial Agents and Chemotherapy* Vol. 54, No. 9, 5 July 2010: 3853-3860. https://doi.org/10.1128/aac.00154-10

VanCompernolle, Scott E. et al. "Antimicrobial Peptides from Amphibian Skin Potently Inhibit

Human Immunodeficiency Virus Infection and Transfer of Virus from Dendritic Cells to T Cells." *Journal of Virology* Vol. 79, No. 18, September 2005: 11598–11606. https://doi.org/10.1128/JVI.79.18.11598-11606.2005

Wang, Suming et al. "Development of a Prosaposin-Derived Therapeuticcyclic Peptide That Targets Ovarian Cancer Via Thetumor Microenvironment." *Science Translational Medicine* Vol. 8, No. 329, 9 Mar 2016: 329ra34. https://doi.org/10.1126/scitranslmed.aad5653

Zhao, Hanjun et al. "A Broad-Spectrum Virus- and Host-Targeting Peptide against Respiratory Viruses Including Influenza Virus and SARS-CoV-2." *Nature Communications* Vol. 11, 25 August 2020. https://doi.org/10.1038/s41467-020-17986-9

Chapter Six

Agyei, Dominic, Ravichandra Potumarthi, and Michael K. Danquah. "Food-Derived Multifunctional Bioactive Proteins and Peptides: Sources and Production," in *Biotechnology of Bioactive Compounds: Sources and Applications.* Eds. Vijai Kumar Gupta et al. John Wiley & Sons, 2015: 483-505.

Boto, Alicia, Jose Manuel Pérez de la Lastra, and Concepción C. González. "The Road from Host-Defense Peptides to a New Generation of Antimicrobial Drugs." Molecules Vol 23,

No. 2, 1 February 2018: 311. https://doi.org/10.3390/molecules23020311

Campione, Elena et al. "Lactoferrin as Protective Natural Barrier of Respiratory and Intestinal Mucosa against Coronavirus Infection and Inflammation." *International Journal of Molecular Sciences* Vol. 21, No. 14, 11 July 2020: 4903. https://doi.org/10.3390/ijms21144903

DeMartini, Alayna. "Higher Carbon Dioxide Levels Prompt More Plant Growth, But Fewer Nutrients." 3 April 2018. Ohio State University College of Food, Agricultural, and Environmental Sciences. https://cfaes.osu.edu/news/articles/higher-carbon-dioxide-levels-prompt-more-plant-growth-fewer-nutrients

Dou, Yan. "The Potential of GHK as an Anti-Aging Peptide." *Aging Pathobiology and Therapeutics* Vol. 2, No. 1, 2020:58-61. https://doi.org/10.31491/APT.2020.03.014

Hemshekhar, Mahadevappa, Vidyanand Anaparti, and Neeloffer Mookherjee. "Functions of Cationic Host Defense Peptides in Immunity." *Pharmaceuticals* Vol. 9, No. 3, September 2016: 40. https://doi.org/10.3390/ph9030040

Ma, Jia et al. "The Positive Effect of Chick Embryo and Nutrient Mixture on Bone Marrow-Derived Mesenchymal Stem Cells from Aging Rats." *Scientific Reports* Vol. 8, Article number: 7051, 04 May 2018. https://doi.org/10.1038/s41598-018-25563-w

Scheer, Roddy and Doug Moss. "Dirt Poor: Have Fruits and Vegetables Become Less Nutritious?" *Scientific American*, 27 April 2011. https://www.scientificamerican.com/article/soil-depletion-and-nutrition-loss/

Steinstraesser, Lars et al. "Host Defense Peptides in Wound Healing." *Molecular Medicine* Vol. 14, 26 March 2008: 528–537. https://doi.org/10.2119/2008-00002.Steinstraesse

Yun, Ye-Rang et al. "Fibroblast Growth Factors: Biology, Function, and Application for Tissue Regeneration." *Journal of Tissue Engineering* Vol. 2010, No. 218142, 7 November 2010. https://doi.org/10.4061/2010/218142

Zhao, Hanjun et al. "A Broad-Spectrum Virus- and Host-Targeting Peptide against Respiratory Viruses Including Influenza Virus and SARS-CoV-2." Nature Communications Vol. 11, 25 August 2020. https://doi.org/10.1038/s41467-020-17986-9

Chapter Seven

Aguirre-Cruz, Gabriel et al. "Collagen Hydrolysates for Skin Protection: Oral Administration and Topical Formulation." *Antioxidants* Vol. 9, No. 2, 22 February 2020: 181. https://doi.org/10.3390/antiox9020181

Bakare, Olalekan Olanrewaju et al. "Dietary Effects of Antimicrobial Peptides in Therapeutics." *All Life*, Vol. 13, No. 1, 17 February 2020:

78-91. https://doi.org/10.1080/26895293.2020.1726826

Dou, Yan et al. "The Potential of GHK as an Anti-Aging Peptide." *Aging Pathologies and Therapeutics* Vol. 2, No. 1, March 2020: 58-61. https://doi.org/10.31491/APT.2020.03.014

Guo, Kaixin et al. "Antioxidant and Anti-Aging Effects of a Sea Cucumber Protein Hydrolyzate and Bioinformatic Characterization of its Composing Peptides." *Food & Function* Vol. 11, 19 May 2020: 5004-5016. https://doi.org/10.1039/D0FO00560F

Jahandideh, Forough and Jianping Wu. "Perspectives on the Potential Benefits of Antihypertensive Peptides towards Metabolic Syndrome." *International Journal of Molecular Sciences* Vol. 21, No. 6, 22 March 2020: 2192. https://doi.org/10.3390/ijms21062192

Kim, Su-Jeong et al. "Mitochondrial-Derived Peptides in Aging and Age-Related Diseases." *GeroScience*, 10 September 2020. https://doi.org/10.1007/s11357-020-00262-5

Laing, Sabrina, et al. "A Dermonutrient Containing Special Collagen Peptides Improves Skin Structure and Function: A Randomized, Placebo-Controlled, Triple-Blind Trial Using Confocal Laser Scanning Microscopy on the Cosmetic Effects and Tolerance of a Drinkable Collagen Supplement." *Journal of Medicinal Food* Vol. 23, No. 2, 31 January 2020. https://doi.org/10.1089/jmf.2019.0197

Lin, Lianzhu et al. "Preparation of Sea Cucumber (*Stichopus Variegates*) Peptide Fraction with Desired Organoleptic Property and its Anti-Aging Activity in Fruit Flies and D-Galactose-Induced Aging Mice." *Journal of Functional Foods* Vol. 69, 10 April 2020. https://doi.org/10.1016/j.jff.2020.103954

Luan, Xin et al. "Cytotoxic and Antitumor Peptides as Novel Chemotherapeutics." *Natural Products Report* 10 August 2020 Aug. Online ahead of print https://doi.org/10.1039/d0np00019a.

Maldonado-Torres, Diego Armando et al. "Modification of Vegetable Proteins to Release Bioactive Peptides Able to Treat Metabolic Syndrome—In Silico Assessment." *Applied Sciences,* Vol. 10, No. 7, 10 April 2020: 2604. https://doi.org/10.3390/app10072604

Moreno-Fernández, Silvia, Marta Garcés-Rimóna and Marta Miguel. "Egg-Derived Peptides and Hydrolysates: A New Bioactive Treasure for Cardiometabolic Diseases." *Trends in Food Science & Technology* Vol. 104, October 2020: 208-218. https://doi.org/10.1016/j.tifs.2020.08.002

Mukherjee, Sumit et al. "Immunoinformatics and Structural Analysis for Identification of Immunodominant Epitopes in SARS-CoV-2 as Potential Vaccine Targets." *Vaccines* Vol. 8, No. 2, 9 June 2020: 290. https://doi.org/10.3390/vaccines8020290

Pan, Xinxing, Juan Xu, and Xuemei Jia. "Research Progress Evaluating the Function and Mechanism of Anti-Tumor Peptides." *Cancer Management and Research* Vol. 12, 16 January 2020: 397–409. https://doi.org/10.2147/CMAR.S232708

Sharkey, Shaun J. et al. "A Narrative Review of the Anti-Hyperglycaemic and Satiating Effects of Fish Protein Hydrolysates and Their Bioactive Peptides." *Molecular Nutrition and Food Research.* Accepted manuscript online: 16 September 2020. https://doi.org/10.1002/mnfr.202000403

Swithenbank, Lucy et al. "Temporin A and Bombinin H2 Antimicrobial Peptides Exhibit Selective Cytotoxicity to Lung Cancer Cells." *Scientifica*, 29 June 2020. https://doi.org/10.1155/2020/3526286

Teng, Qiu-Xu et al. "Anticancer and Multidrug Resistance-Reversing Activities of Novel Antimicrobial Peptides [Abstract]." Proceedings of the Annual Meeting of the American Association for Cancer Research, April 27-28 and June 22-24, 2020, Philadelphia (PA). *Cancer Research* Vol. 20, No. 16 Supplement, August 2020. https://doi.org/10.1158/1538-7445.AM2020-3006

Tornesello, Anna Lucia. "Antimicrobial Peptides as Anticancer Agents: Functional Properties and Biological Activities." *Molecules* Vol.25,

No. 12, 19 June 2020: 2850. https://doi.org/10.3390/molecules25122850

Xie, Mingfeng, Dijia Liu and Yufeng Yang. "Anti-Cancer Peptides: Classification, Mechanism of Action, Reconstruction and Modification." *Open Biology* Vol. 10, No. 7, 22 July 2020. https://doi.org/10.1098/rsob.200004

Yen, Kelvin et al. "The Mitochondrial Derived Peptide Humanin is a Regulator of Lifespan and Healthspan." *Aging* Vol. 12, No. 12, 23 June 2020: 11185—11199. https://doi.org/10.18632/aging.103534

—— et al. "Humanin Prevents Age-Related Cognitive Decline in Mice and is Associated with Improved Cognitive Age in Humans." *Scientific Reports* Vol. 8, 21 September 2018: Article number 14212. https://doi.org/10.1038/s41598-018-32616-7